THE AMERICAN FOUNTAIN OF YOUTH

SECRETS OF A LONG & JOYFUL LIFE

TABLE OF CONTENT

CHAPTER ONE
Preparing for a Long and Joyful Life

In this opening chapter, we embark on a voyage into the profound exploration of a life filled with purpose, fulfillment, and boundless joy. Life is a journey, and how we navigate it shapes our destinies. This book will serve as your compass, guiding you through the seas of existence, and offering insights, tools, and wisdom to help you chart a course towards a long and joyful life. Together, we will discover the keys to not only prolonging our time on this planet but also savoring every moment of it. So, prepare to embark on this adventure, for the voyage of a lifetime awaits.

The "American Fountain of Youth" is a metaphorical concept that symbolizes the idea of maintaining youthfulness, vitality, and a high quality of life as one grows older. It draws inspiration from the mythical Fountain of Youth, which, according to legends, had the power to restore youth and grant immortality to those who drank from it.

In the context of your book, "American Fountain of Youth" represents a mindset and a way of living that can help individuals achieve a long and joyful life. Here are some key aspects of the power of the "American Fountain of Youth":

1. Positive Aging: It encourages individuals to embrace the process of aging with a positive attitude. Instead of fearing or resisting getting older, the concept promotes the idea that aging can be a rewarding experience.

2. Health and Wellness: The "American Fountain of Youth" emphasizes the importance of maintaining good physical and mental health through a healthy lifestyle. This includes aspects like proper nutrition, regular exercise, and stress management.

3. Mindset and Attitude: A youthful mindset is seen as a powerful tool for longevity and happiness. It encourages people to maintain a curious, open-minded, and optimistic outlook on life.

4. Pursuit of Passions: Engaging in activities that one is passionate about is considered a vital component of the "American Fountain of Youth." It's about finding joy and purpose in one's hobbies, interests, and creative endeavors.

5. Social Connections: Building and nurturing positive relationships with others is believed to be a key to a joyful life. This includes maintaining strong connections with family and friends and fostering a sense of community and belonging.

6. Adaptability: The concept promotes adaptability and resilience in the face of life's challenges. It suggests that those who can adapt to change and learn from their experiences are more likely to lead fulfilling lives.

7. Life-Long Learning: Continuous learning and personal growth are valued elements of the "American Fountain of Youth." It encourages individuals to stay curious and continue acquiring new knowledge and skills.

8. Giving Back: Contributing to the well-being of others and giving back to the community is seen as a source of fulfillment. It suggests that acts of kindness and philanthropy can add meaning to one's life.

In essence, the "American Fountain of Youth" is a way of life that focuses on proactively nurturing physical, mental, and emotional well-being while maintaining a positive and purposeful mindset. It's not about seeking eternal youth but about aging gracefully and joyfully, making the most of each stage of life. This concept reminds individuals that they have the power to shape their aging journey and live a fulfilling life, regardless of their age.

The promise of a joyful life is a powerful and optimistic vision of what life can be when one consciously pursues happiness, fulfillment, and contentment. It's the idea that by making deliberate choices and adopting certain attitudes and behaviors, individuals can significantly enhance their overall quality of life. Here are some key elements that constitute the promise of a joyful life:

1. Happiness and Contentment: At the heart of this promise is the pursuit of happiness and contentment. It acknowledges that true joy comes from within and can be cultivated through positive thoughts, experiences, and relationships.

2. Purpose and Meaning: A joyful life often involves a sense of purpose and meaning. It's about feeling that one's life has value and that one's actions and contributions matter.

3. Positive Relationships: Strong, supportive, and loving relationships with family and friends are essential for a joyful life. These connections provide emotional support, companionship, and a sense of belonging.

4. Gratitude: Practicing gratitude and appreciating the small and big blessings in life is a fundamental aspect of a joyful life. Gratitude helps shift focus away from what's lacking and toward what's present and positive.

5. Fulfilling Activities: Engaging in activities, hobbies, or work that one is passionate about can bring immense joy. These pursuits provide a sense of accomplishment and personal satisfaction.

6. Emotional Resilience: The ability to bounce back from adversity and cope with life's challenges is crucial for a joyful life. Resilience helps individuals maintain a positive outlook, even in difficult times.

7. Self-Care: Taking care of one's physical and mental health is part of the promise of a joyful life. Self-care practices, such as exercise, meditation, and relaxation, contribute to overall well-being.

8. Balance: Achieving a balance between various aspects of life, such as work, leisure, and personal time, is important for happiness. A balanced life allows for personal growth and enjoyment.

9. Optimism: An optimistic outlook on life can help individuals overcome obstacles and view setbacks as opportunities for growth.

10. Continuous Learning: A commitment to lifelong learning and personal growth is a hallmark of a joyful life. It fosters a sense of curiosity and self-improvement.

11. Kindness and Generosity: Acts of kindness and generosity, whether toward others or oneself, are associated with increased happiness and a sense of fulfillment.

12. Living in the Present: The promise of a joyful life often encourages individuals to be fully present in the moment, rather than dwelling on the past or worrying about the future.

In essence, the promise of a joyful life is a belief that individuals have the power to shape their happiness and fulfillment. It's a commitment to making choices and cultivating habits that lead to a life filled with positivity, purpose, and well-being. While challenges and difficulties may arise, the promise of a joyful life suggests that with the right mindset and actions, one can navigate life's ups and downs with grace and resilience.

Wisdom Words:

"Embrace the gift of each day with a heart full of gratitude, a mind open to learning, and a spirit eager to share kindness. In these simple yet profound acts, you'll uncover the secret to a lifetime of joy."

Call to Action:

As you close this book and embark on your journey towards a long and joyful life, remember that the power to shape your destiny lies within you. I encourage you to take the following actions today:

1. Set Clear Goals: Define your aspirations and set achievable goals for your future. Write them down and create a plan to work towards them.

2. Practice Gratitude: Start a daily gratitude journal. Write down three things you're grateful for each day, no matter how small or significant.

3. Nurture Relationships: Reach out to a loved one you haven't connected with in a while. Strengthen your bonds with family and friends.

4. Engage in a Passion: Dedicate time to a hobby or interest that brings you joy. Rekindle your passions.

5. Take Care of Your Health: Commit to a healthier lifestyle. Incorporate regular exercise and balanced nutrition into your daily routine.

6. Learn Something New: Identify a subject or skill you've always wanted to explore and take the first steps toward learning it.

7. Give Back: Find a way to give back to your community or a cause you're passionate about. Acts of kindness make a difference.

8. Stay Present: Practice mindfulness. Spend a few moments each day living in the present, appreciating the beauty of now.

Remember, a joyful life is not a destination but a continuous journey. Seize each day as an opportunity to shape your destiny and find happiness in the smallest of moments. Your life is your masterpiece, and you are the artist. Paint it with the vibrant colors of joy, purpose, and fulfillment."

The Search for Eternal Knowledge

The eternal pursuit of youth and the key to a long and happy life continue to be subjects of intrigue in a society where it feels as though time is flying by. The pursuit of life and happiness has captivated human imagination for millennia, from the legends surrounding the fabled Fountain of Youth to the most recent scientific discoveries in anti-aging research.

We start our voyage with a thorough investigation of this age-old interest, one that takes us through the archives of science, mythology, history, and the collective knowledge of many cultures. We welcome you to set out on a personal quest with "The American Fountain of Youth," a mission to discover the mysteries that will enable you to live a life full of vitality, meaning, and fulfillment.

There has never been a greater need for this mission. With an increasing life expectancy comes the task of living life to the fullest as well as the gift of more years. We now possess the information and resources necessary to not only live longer lives but also to improve the quality of those extra years thanks to developments in science, medicine, and our understanding of wellbeing.

This book serves as a multifaceted guide to the secrets of happiness and longevity, acting as your compass on this incredible trip. We'll explore the science behind aging, the importance of diet and exercise, mental health, and heredity. The experiences of those who reside in "Blue Zones," where people live longer, healthier lives, will teach us valuable lessons. We'll examine the myths and fallacies surrounding aging and the fountain of youth, separating fact from fiction.

The upcoming chapters will present a thorough road map, along with useful tips and doable actions for people of all ages. This book will provide you with the tools to make wise decisions for a happier, healthier life, from fitness and nutrition advice to the knowledge of accepting aging with grace.

We want you to approach this journey with an open mind and an open heart as we set out on it together. Every chapter in the trip toward a future full of the promise of enduring vitality and happiness is a step toward the goal of living a long and happy life.

Now turn the page and let's embark on this amazing adventure to find the American Fountain of Youth and all the mysteries it can reveal to you and your family.

CHAPTER TWO

Historical Perspectives: Legends and Myths of the Fountain of Youth

In this chapter, we will step back in time to explore the captivating tales and enduring myths surrounding the elusive Fountain of Youth. These stories, passed down through generations, have left an indelible mark on our collective imagination. We will unravel the origins of these legends, examining their cultural significance and their enduring impact on the quest for eternal youth. By delving into the historical perspectives surrounding the Fountain of Youth, we will gain a deeper understanding of how human aspirations for longevity have been shaped by the narratives of the past.

The Myth of Ponce de León and the Fountain of Youth

In the early 16th century, the Spanish explorer Juan Ponce de León set sail for the newly discovered lands of the Americas. He is often associated with the quest for the Fountain of Youth, a legendary spring said to have the power to restore youth and vitality to those who drink from its waters.

According to the myth, Ponce de León heard of the Fountain's existence from the indigenous people he encountered in Florida. They told him of a miraculous spring hidden deep within the lush forests, a place where the waters possessed the magical ability to reverse the aging process. Driven by the allure of eternal youth, Ponce de León embarked on a relentless search for this mythical source of rejuvenation.

His expedition took him to various parts of Florida, and while he encountered beautiful natural springs and water sources, the legendary Fountain of Youth remained elusive. Despite his relentless efforts, Ponce de León never discovered the fabled spring, and the quest for eternal youth remained unfulfilled.

In reality, Ponce de León's explorations were more focused on territorial expansion and wealth, and the idea of him seeking the Fountain of Youth was largely a later myth. However, the tale of his quest has

Become an enduring part of folklore, symbolizing humanity's age-old desire for immortality and the pursuit of a long and vibrant life.

The myth of Ponce de León and the Fountain of Youth continues to captivate our imagination, serving as a reminder of the profound, timeless yearning for everlasting youth and the secrets it may hold.

The Myth of Ponce de León and the Fountain of Youth

Tales of sacred, restorative waters existed well before the birth of Spanish conquistador Juan Ponce de León around 1474. Alexander the Great, for example, was said to have come across a healing "river of paradise" in the fourth century B.C., and similar legends cropped up in such disparate locations as the Canary Islands, Japan, Polynesia, and England. During the Middle Ages, some Europeans even believed in the mythical king Prester John, whose kingdom allegedly contained a fountain of youth and a river of gold. "You could trace that up until today," said Ryan K. Smith, a history professor at Virginia Commonwealth University. "People are still touting miracle cures and miracle waters."

Spanish sources asserted that the Taino Indians of the Caribbean also spoke of a magic fountain and rejuvenating river that existed somewhere north of Cuba. These rumors conceivably reached the ears of Ponce de León, who is thought to have accompanied Christopher Columbus on his second voyage to the New World in 1493. After helping to brutally crush a Taino rebellion on Hispaniola in 1504, Ponce de León was granted a provincial governorship and hundreds of acres of land, where he used forced Indian labor to raise crops and livestock. In 1508 he received royal permission to colonize San Juan Bautista (now Puerto Rico). He became the island's first governor a year later but was soon pushed out in a power struggle with Christopher Columbus' son Diego.

Having remained in the good graces of King Ferdinand, Ponce de León received a contract in 1512 to explore and settle an island called Bimini. Nowhere in either this contract or a follow-up contract was the Fountain of Youth mentioned. By contrast, specific instructions were given for subjugating the Indians and divvying up any gold found. Although he may have claimed to know certain "secrets," Ponce de León likewise never brought up the fountain in his known correspondence with Ferdinand.

"What Ponce is looking for is islands that will become part of what he hopes will be a profitable new governorship," said J. Michael Francis, a history professor at the University of South Florida St. Petersburg. "From everything I can gather, he was not at all interested or believed that he would find some kind of miraculous spring or lake or body of water." At least one historian suggests that perhaps Ferdinand, who had recently married a woman 35 years his junior, told Ponce de León to keep his eye out for it. But other experts dispute this.

Either way, Ponce de León set sail in March 1513 with three ships. According to early historians, he anchored off the eastern coast of Florida on April 2 and came ashore a day later, choosing the name "La Florida" in part because it was the Easter season (Pascua Florida in Spanish). Ponce de León then journeyed down through the Florida Keys and up the western coast, where he skirmished with Indians, before beginning a roundabout journey back to Puerto Rico. Along the way, he purportedly discovered the Gulf Stream, which proved to be the fastest route for sailing back to Europe.

Eight years later, Ponce de León returned to Florida's southwestern coast in an attempt to establish a colony, but he was mortally wounded by an Indian arrow. Just before leaving, he sent letters to his new king, Charles V, and the future Pope Adrian VI. Once again, the explorer made no mention of the Fountain of Youth, focusing instead on his desire to settle the land, spread Christianity, and discover whether Florida was an island or a peninsula. No log of either voyage has survived, and no archaeological footprint has ever been uncovered.

Nonetheless, historians began linking Ponce de León with the Fountain of Youth not long after his death. In 1535 Gonzalo Fernández de Oviedo y Valdés accused Ponce de León of seeking the fountain to cure his sexual impotence. "He was being discredited [as] an idiot and weakling," Smith explained. "This is machismo culture in Spain at the height of the Counter-Reformation." The accusation is almost certainly untrue, Smith added, since Ponce de León fathered several children and was under 40 years old at the time of his first expedition.

Hernando de Escalante Fontaneda, who lived with Indians in Florida for many years after surviving a shipwreck, also derided Ponce de León in his 1575 memoir, saying it was a cause for merriment that he sought out the Fountain of Youth. One of the next authors to weigh in was Antonio de Herrera y Tordesillas, the Spanish king's chief historian of the Indies. In 1601 he penned a detailed and widely read account of Ponce de León's first voyage. Although Herrera only referred to the Fountain of Youth in passing, writing that it turned "old men to boys," he helped solidify it in the public's imagination. "They are more entertainment than attempts to write a true history," Francis said of these works.

The Fountain of Youth legend was now alive and well. It did not gain much traction in the United States, however, until the Spanish ceded Florida in 1819. Famous writers of the time such as Washington Irving then began portraying Ponce de León as hapless and vain. Artists also got in on the act, including Thomas Moran, who painted an oversize canvas of Ponce de León meeting with Indians.

By the early 20th century, a statue of the explorer had been placed in the central plaza of Florida's oldest city, St. Augustine, and a nearby tourist attraction pretended to be the actual Fountain of Youth. To this day, tens of thousands of visitors come every year to sample the sulfur-smelling well water. "It does not taste good," said Smith, who worked there for four days in college. "Imagine what you would think the Fountain of Youth would taste like. It doesn't taste like that." Meanwhile, some grade school textbooks continue to present Ponce de León's search for the fountain as a historical fact.

In 2013, Ponce de León was back in the spotlight. In celebration of the 500th anniversary of his landing, reenactments took place in St. Augustine and Melbourne Beach, Florida, both of which claim to be the site where he first dropped anchor. There was also a Catholic mass in St. Augustine featuring a replica of the 15th-century font used to baptize him in Spain and a mass In Melbourne Beach, along with the unveiling of more statues and a commemorative stamp.

What would Ponce de León make of all this attention, not all of it positive? "My take on that is that no publicity is bad publicity," Smith said. "He's a household name, and maybe in the end that's what he was looking for."

In this chapter, we've journeyed through the annals of time to explore the fascinating myth of Ponce de León and the Fountain of Youth. This legendary tale, though rooted in the age of exploration, continues to resonate with us today. It serves as a vivid example of how our pursuit of a longer, more joyful life has been colored by the captivating narratives of the past.

As we close the pages of this chapter, we reflect on how the myth of Ponce de León's quest mirrors the timeless human quest for eternal youth. While the elusive Fountain of Youth may remain hidden in the mists of myth and legend, the longing for vitality, health, and the preservation of youth endures as a shared aspiration.

Yet, as we turn to the following chapters, we'll transition from the realm of myth and history to the domain of science, exploring the biological and practical aspects of longevity. The stories of the past will continue to inform our journey, reminding us that the quest for a long and joyful life has been a human endeavor for centuries. It's a quest that transcends time and culture, and it's a journey that we are on together, seeking to uncover the enduring secrets of a life well-lived.

The Myth of TithonusIn

In Greek mythology, Tithonus was a mortal prince of Troy, known for his striking handsomeness. His story is often associated with the concept of immortality without eternal youth. Tithonus was the son of King Laomedon of Troy, and he caught the eye of Eos, the goddess of the dawn. Eos, captivated by Tithonus's beauty, carried him away to the eastern edges of the world, and they fell in love. In her infatuation, Eos begged Zeus to grant Tithonus immortality, desiring to keep him with her forever. Zeus granted her request, but Eos made a critical oversight. She forgot to ask for eternal youth for Tithonus along with immortality. As a result, Tithonus continued to age, growing older and more frail with each passing year, while Eos remained eternally youthful. Tithonus's immortality became a curse. He aged until he was bent and feeble, unable to move or speak coherently. He became a mere whisper of his former self, trapped in a body that continued to deteriorate. His condition was pitiable, and he could not escape the passage of time. Eos, deeply saddened by her beloved's fate, placed Tithonus in a room where he could make no sound, preserving his existence but unable to relieve his suffering. This sad tale of Tithonus serves as a poignant reminder that immortality without eternal youth can lead to a life of endless and unbearable agony. In the end, Eos's love for Tithonus, while well-intentioned, resulted in a tragedy of unending senescence, highlighting the importance of maintaining both youth and immortality in the pursuit of a long and joyful life.

:

The Quest for the Philosopher's Stone

The Quest for the Philosopher's Stone is a tale deeply rooted in medieval alchemy, where the pursuit of transmutation, immortality, and the secrets of eternal youth were central themes.

In the heart of the Middle Ages, alchemists toiled tirelessly in their laboratories, seeking the elusive Philosopher's Stone. This legendary substance, it was believed, possessed extraordinary powers. It was said to have the ability to transmute base metals, like lead, into precious ones, such as gold. But the allure of the Philosopher's Stone extended far beyond mere material wealth.

Alchemy was both a physical and spiritual pursuit. The Philosopher's Stone was thought to be a key to eternal life and youth. It was believed that its discovery would not only allow the transmutation of base metals but also the transformation of the alchemist, granting them longevity and a rejuvenated, youthful existence.

Legends of the stone's existence and magical properties were widespread. Alchemists from Europe to the Middle East dedicated their lives to uncovering its secrets. They documented their experiments, sought hidden knowledge in ancient texts, and sought divine inspiration to unlock the mysteries of the universe.

The search for the Philosopher's Stone became a symbol of the human quest for transcendence—a pursuit that blended the material and the spiritual, the scientific and the mystical. Although the Philosopher's Stone was never found in the literal sense, the alchemical tradition contributed to the development of modern chemistry and the search for longevity.

As we explore the historical roots of the quest for eternal youth, the story of the Philosopher's Stone stands as a testament to the enduring human fascination with immortality, the secrets of youth, and the profound transformations of both the material and the self in the quest for a longer and more joyful life.

Chinese Legends of Longevity

Chinese culture has a rich tradition of stories and legends centered around the quest for longevity and the secrets to a long, healthy life. These legends often feature revered figures who achieved remarkable longevity or possessed the wisdom to guide others on the path to a fulfilling and enduring existence. Here are a few notable Chinese legends related to longevity:

1. The Eight Immortals (Ba Xian): The Eight Immortals are a group of legendary figures in Chinese mythology, each possessing unique powers and qualities. They are known for their immortality and their ability to bestow blessings upon those they encounter. These immortals have been celebrated for centuries and symbolize various aspects of longevity, wisdom, and happiness.

2. The Peaches of Immortality: In Chinese mythology, there is a heavenly orchard where the Peaches of Immortality grow. Consuming these peaches grants longevity and eternal youth. The Jade Emperor, a high-ranking deity

in Chinese folklore, hosts a feast featuring these peaches, and those who partake are said to gain immortality.

3. The Tale of Zhang Guolao: Zhang Guolao is one of the Eight Immortals and is often depicted as an old man riding a mule backward. He possesses the power of immortality and is known for his ability to bring back the dead. His legend emphasizes the importance of wise and virtuous living for a long life.

4. The Legend of Xu Fu: Xu Fu was a historical figure sent by Emperor Qin Shi Huang in search of the elixir of life. He embarked on a legendary voyage to find the fabled elixir and extend the emperor's life. Although he did not return, his story highlights the quest for longevity in ancient China.

5. The Peach Blossom Spring: While not directly related to longevity, the Peach Blossom Spring is a famous Chinese fable about a hidden utopia. It represents the ideal of a peaceful and harmonious life, which is often associated with a long and content existence.

These Chinese legends are woven into the cultural fabric of China and continue to influence the pursuit of longevity and happiness in Chinese society. They convey the enduring human aspiration for a life of health, wisdom, and immortality, and they offer valuable insights for those seeking the secrets of a long and joyful life.

The Algonquian Legend of Manabozho

The Algonquian people, a group of Native American tribes from the northeastern United States and eastern Canada, have a rich oral tradition filled with legends and myths, including those featuring Manabozho, a prominent figure in their folklore.

Manabozho, also known as Nanabozho or EvenManabush, is a cultural hero and trickster figure who plays a central role in Algonquian mythology. He is a shape-shifter, cultural creator, and teacher. While Manabozho's stories vary among different Algonquian tribes, here is a general overview of the legend:

Birth and Early Adventures:

Manabozho is often said to have been born to a mortal woman and the West Wind. His birth is shrouded in mystery and supernatural events. As a young boy, he displayed a mischievous and curious nature, often engaging in playful antics and pranks.

The Great Flood:

One of Manabozho's most well-known feats was his role in saving the world from a great flood. He was warned of the impending deluge by a vision and warned the animals and people to build a raft to survive the flood. He guided them to safety and played a crucial role in restoring life on Earth after the waters receded.

Teaching and Cultural Contributions:

Manabozho is revered as a teacher and cultural hero who imparted valuable knowledge and wisdom to the Algonquian people. He taught them essential skills, such as hunting, fishing, and survival techniques. Manabozho also played a role in explaining the natural world, creation myths, and tribal customs.

Trickster Adventures:

Manabozho is also a trickster figure. He often used his cunning and humor to outsmart rivals and adversaries. These trickster tales serve as both entertainment and moral lessons, highlighting the importance of wit and resourcefulness.

Manabozho's adventures and teachings in Algonquian folklore are diverse and vary among the different tribes, but the common theme is his significance as a cultural figure and his role in guiding and shaping the lives of the Algonquian people.

The Algonquian legend of Manabozho is a testament to the cultural richness and depth of Native American folklore, emphasizing the importance of knowledge, resourcefulness, and the interconnectedness of humans and the natural world.

The Search for the Holy Grail

The Holy Grail is a sacred relic with profound significance in Christian tradition. It is believed to be the cup used by Jesus Christ during the Last Supper, and later, it was said to have caught His blood during the Crucifixion. In medieval Arthurian legends, the quest for the Holy Grail becomes a central and symbolic theme.

The story begins with King Arthur and his Knights of the Round Table. The knights, known for their chivalry and honor, embark on a quest to find the Holy Grail, which is thought to possess miraculous powers, including the ability to heal and sustain life.

The quest for the Holy Grail is intertwined with various adventures and challenges faced by the knights. Sir Percival, Sir Galahad, Sir Lancelot, and other renowned knights are among those who undertake this noble pursuit. Each knight must prove their worthiness and righteousness to even catch a glimpse of the sacred relic.

The knights' journeys take them through enchanting forests, treacherous mountains, and mystical lands. They encounter strange characters, including the Fisher King, who guards the Grail and is often wounded and in need of healing. The knights face moral dilemmas, personal trials, and the temptations of the flesh as they strive to remain pure and virtuous on their quest.

Sir Galahad, often portrayed as the purest of the knights, ultimately achieves the Grail and attains a vision of divine glory. His exceptional virtue and unwavering faith make him the chosen one to witness the Holy Grail's true essence.

The quest for the Holy Grail is not just a physical journey; it's a spiritual one that tests the knights' character, resolve, and piety. It represents the human quest for spiritual enlightenment, purity, and communion with the divine.

The Grail's ultimate significance and the interpretation of the story can vary, but the enduring appeal of the legend lies in its portrayal of the noble pursuit of higher ideals, spiritual awakening, and the eternal search for that which is sacred and transcendent.

The story of the search for the Holy Grail has been a source of inspiration for countless writers, artists, and filmmakers, and it continues to capture the imagination with its blend of chivalry, mysticism, and profound meaning.

The "Epic of Gilgamesh

 Is an ancient Mesopotamian narrative, often regarded as one of the earliest surviving works of literature. It tells the story of Gilgamesh, a historical figure who ruled the Sumerian city of Uruk around 2700 BC. Here is a condensed version of the epic:

The Epic of Gilgamesh

Prologue:

The epic begins by introducing Gilgamesh, a king who is part god and part man. He is a powerful and arrogant ruler, but his people cry out to the gods for relief from his oppressive behavior. In response, the gods create Enkidu, a wild man, to challenge and humble Gilgamesh.

Meeting Enkidu:

Enkidu lives in the wilderness, away from human civilization, until he is tamed by a temple prostitute. He learns the ways of human society and becomes more like a man. Enkidu's connection with nature and the animals is a central theme of the story.

The Clash of Titans:

Enkidu is sent to Uruk, where he confronts Gilgamesh. The two engage in a mighty battle, but eventually, Gilgamesh prevails. Their confrontation leads to mutual respect, and they become close friends.

The Quest for Immortality:

Gilgamesh and Enkidu set out on a heroic quest. They decide to journey to the Cedar Forest to defeat Humbaba, a monstrous guardian. After their victory, the goddess Ishtar proposes marriage to Gilgamesh, but he rejects her, invoking her anger. As a consequence, the gods decide that one of the two friends must die. Enkidu falls ill and eventually dies, leaving Gilgamesh devastated.

Gilgamesh's Grief:

Gilgamesh is consumed by grief and a fear of his mortality. He embarks on a new quest, this time to find Utnapishtim, a man who survived a great flood and gained immortality. Utnapishtim tells Gilgamesh the story of the flood and offers a challenge to stay awake for a week, which Gilgamesh fails.

The Return to Uruk:

Gilgamesh ultimately realizes that true immortality is beyond his reach. He returns to Uruk, a changed man. He has learned to accept the limitations of mortality and to appreciate the value of human life. The epic ends with Gilgamesh becoming a wise and just ruler, celebrated for his achievements and contributions to his city.

The "Epic of Gilgamesh" explores profound themes such as the nature of friendship, the human quest for immortality, and the acceptance of mortality. It is a story of personal growth, transformation, and the pursuit of wisdom that has resonated through the ages and continues to be a cherished work of ancient literature.

The myth of the Elixir of Life, often associated with alchemy and various cultures, is a tale of a substance or potion that grants immortality, eternal youth, or profound longevity. While the specifics of the myth vary across cultures and periods,

The Myth of the Elixir of Life

In ancient times, there existed a legendary Elixir of Life, a potion said to grant those who consumed it the gift of immortality, eternal youth, and unending vitality. The search for this elixir was a quest pursued by sages, alchemists, and ambitious individuals throughout history.

The Elixir was often associated with the Philosopher's Stone, another mythical substance sought after by alchemists. The Philosopher's Stone was believed to have the power to transmute base metals into gold, but it was also thought to be a crucial ingredient in the creation of the Elixir of Life.

The recipe for the Elixir of Life was a closely guarded secret, handed down through generations of alchemists. It typically required the use of rare and mystical ingredients, intricate procedures, and often a deep understanding of esoteric knowledge.

Across different cultures and regions, various stories emerged about individuals who claimed to have found the Elixir of Life or those who sought it desperately. Chinese, Indian, European, and Middle Eastern cultures all have their versions of this myth.

In Chinese mythology, the search for the Elixir of Life was central to the quests of many emperors and legendary figures. In India, the concept of "amrita" is similar, representing a nectar of immortality. In Europe, alchemists like Nicholas Flamel were famous for their quest to discover the Elixir of Life, which was thought to endow them with not only immortality but also great wisdom.

While the Elixir of Life remained elusive and the Philosopher's Stone was never found in reality, the pursuit of these mythical substances had a profound impact on the development of alchemy, early chemistry, and the search for the secrets of longevity.

The enduring fascination with the Elixir of Life represents humanity's deep-seated desire to conquer mortality and enjoy a life of perpetual youth and vitality. While the elixir remains a mythical concept, the quest for health, longevity, and well-being continues to be a fundamental aspiration in human culture and history.

Certainly, several notable individuals in the modern era achieved extraordinary longevity. Here are a few examples:

1. Jeanne Calment (1875-1997): Jeanne Calment, a French woman, holds the record for the longest confirmed human lifespan, living to the age of 122. Her remarkable longevity has been extensively documented, and she remains an iconic figure in the study of aging.

2. Sarah Knauss (1880-1999): Sarah Knauss, an American woman, lived to be 119 years old. She held the title of the world's oldest living person for some time before her passing.

3. Jiroemon Kimura (1897-2013): Jiroemon Kimura, a Japanese man, became the world's oldest living person and the oldest man in recorded history, living to the age of 116. His longevity was attributed to his healthy lifestyle, including a diet rich in vegetables.

4. Misao Okawa (1898-2015): Misao Okawa, also from Japan, was the world's oldest living person before her death at the age of 117. She credited her long life to eating plenty of sushi and sleeping well.

5. Emma Morano (1899-2017): Emma Morano, an Italian woman, held the title of the world's oldest living person before her passing at the age of 117. She attributed her longevity to a diet rich in eggs and a stress-free life.

6. Violet Brown (1900-2017): Violet Brown from Jamaica became the world's oldest living person after the death of Emma Morano. She lived to be 117 years old and passed away in 2017.

7. Kane Tanaka (1903-Present): Kane Tanaka, a Japanese woman, is currently one of the oldest living people in the world. She was recognized as the world's oldest living person at one point and is known for her love of board games and sweets.

These individuals serve as inspiring examples of the potential for exceptional longevity in the modern era. While genetics may play a role, their stories also emphasize the importance of a healthy lifestyle, including a balanced diet, regular exercise, and positive mental well-being.

In this chapter, we've explored a tapestry of historical legends and myths, each offering its unique take on the timeless human fascination with eternal youth and longevity. From the alchemical quests for the Philosopher's Stone to the sagas of legendary figures like Tithonus and Manabozho, these stories remind us of the enduring quest for life's most precious gift – time.

These legends, originating from diverse cultures and eras, share a common thread – the unquenchable human desire for longevity, health, and vitality. As we step into the following chapters, we move from the world of myth and history into the realm of science and practice, where we'll seek practical knowledge and insights to unlock the secrets of a long and joyful life.

The legends we've explored serve as a bridge between ancient wisdom and contemporary understanding, illuminating the path ahead. The quest for a fulfilling and enduring existence continues, and in the chapters to come, we'll dive deeper into the modern approaches and strategies that guide us in this timeless pursuit. Historical Perspectives: Legends and Myths of the Fountain of Yout

Chapter Three

The Science of Aging

Welcome to Chapter 3 of our journey, where we venture into the heart of longevity science. In this chapter, we embark on an exploration of the intricate and fascinating world of aging and the biology behind the quest for a longer, healthier life.

As we move from the legends and myths of the past, we transition to the realm of modern understanding. Here, we will uncover the profound secrets hidden within our genes, cells, and bodies—secrets that hold the promise of extending our vitality and well-being.

This chapter is a gateway to the exciting world of longevity research, offering insights into the factors that influence the aging process and the mechanisms that can slow it down. We'll learn how our genetic makeup, lifestyle choices, and the environment interact to shape our journey through time.

The Science of Aging is a voyage of discovery, a quest to unravel the mysteries of our biology. Together, we'll dive deep into the scientific foundations of longevity and equip ourselves with knowledge that can empower us to lead not just longer lives, but fuller and healthier ones. Join us on this compelling journey into the intricacies of our biological clock and the pathways to a life brimming with vitality.

Understanding the Odd Science of Aging

Evolutionary considerations suggest aging is caused not by active gene programming but by evolved limitations in somatic maintenance, resulting in a build-up of damage. Ecological factors such as hazard rates and food availability influence the trade-offs between investing in growth, reproduction, and somatic survival, explaining why species evolved different life spans and why the aging rate can sometimes be altered, for example, by dietary restriction. To understand the cell and molecular basis of aging is to unravel the multiplicity of mechanisms causing damage to accumulate and the complex array of systems working to keep damage at bay.

Aging is arguably the most familiar yet least well-understood aspect of human biology. Each of us quickly acquires knowledge of the aging process, first by observing what it does to others and then by experiencing its effects ourselves. Most can offer some kind of theory as to why aging exists and how it is caused. However, most of these ideas are substantially, if not entirely, incorrect. In particular, there is a widespread but erroneous tendency to regard aging as programmed. As we shall see, there is scant evidence for the existence of such a program, and there are powerful arguments why it should not exist. Part of the oddity of aging science thus derives from the fact that we must begin by dismantling important preconceptions about why aging occurs.

The second oddity about aging is its inherent complexity. Almost every aspect of an organism's phenotype undergoes modification with aging, and this phenomenological complexity has led, over the years, to a bewildering proliferation of ideas about specific cellular and molecular causes. An attempt by Medvedev, 1990 to rationalize the multiplicity of hypotheses resulted in a listing of more than 300 "theories" of aging. Fortunately, recent advances have resulted in significant simplification of the theoretical underpinnings of aging research, and this, combined with the greatly increased power of experimental techniques to investigate the phenomenological complexities of the senescent phenotype, has helped clear a path toward unraveling the workings of the aging process. Nevertheless, the intrinsic complexity of aging remains a significant challenge to understanding how aging is caused.

Because aging occurs for nonintuitive reasons and unfolds in complex ways, theory plays an unusually pivotal role in its research. This review examines and critically assesses the current framework of ideas about why and how aging happens. It then considers some of how the aging rate can be modified, and it concludes by examining some of the instances that push the boundary of our understanding of the aging process.

Setting the Stage

In recent years the field of longevity has exploded, with scientists making significant breakthroughs in understanding how we can live longer, healthier lives.

As these scientists continue to uncover how and why we age, their research suggests that aging may be a somewhat modifiable process. Science-backed interventions show promise in slowing down the aging process and increasing lifespan. According to these experts, aging may not be inevitable.

What is aging and when does it start?

Aging is a gradual decrease in function due to the accumulation of cellular damage. More broadly, aging is the culmination of the physiological changes that occur over our lifespans. While some of these changes are seemingly harmless (like graying hair and wrinkles) others have a more profound impact—affecting aspects of health like mobility, bone strength, and disease susceptibility.

Aging is a complex, non-linear process that is considered to begin in the fourth decade of life, between the ages of 30-39 years. However, each person ages at a unique rate. Some people maintain their mental capacity and stamina well into their later years, whereas others begin exhibiting signs of aging as early as their mid-20s. While genetics and biology play a key role, the rate of aging is also significantly impacted by behavioral and psychological factors including diet, physical activity, smoking status, stress levels, sleep patterns, and social connections.

Why do we age?

Initially, aging was believed to be an evolutionary benefit to the human species—aging and eventual death prevented overcrowding and allowed for the survival of beneficial genetic traits. But, advances in research have made it clear that this complex, multifaceted process cannot be attributed to a singular cause. Rather the more widely Accepted explanation is that aging is the result of multiple genetic, biological, and environmental processes combining, interacting, and overlapping with each other on a variety of levels.

Theories on aging

Given the inherent complexities of aging, scientists have theorized for years about the exact mechanisms behind the process as they seek to understand the cause, effect, and what keeps it at bay. At one point, over 300 different theories attempted to explain the phenomenon.

Advances in research geared towards unraveling the process have led to two prevailing categories of aging: programmed theories of aging and damage theories of aging.

Programmed theory of aging

Programmed theories center around the notion that aging is an innate part of biology. Cells are programmed to decay and deliberately deteriorate in function over time. In other words, cells have a finite lifespan.

Genetic theory: According to this theory, aging is caused by switching 'on' and 'off' certain genes.

Endocrine theory: This theory links the pace of aging with hormone levels. Levels of hormones that control processes like blood sugar regulation decline with age and cause dysregulation in cellular processes.

Immunological theory: This theory is based on the fact that the immune system is programmed to peak during adolescence and decline over time, resulting in increased susceptibility to illness and disease.

Damage theory of aging

Damage theories of aging view aging not as inherent, but rather, as an accumulation of damage caused by environmental factors. According to this theory, wear and tear are the main drivers of aging.

Wear and tear theory: This theory suggests that cells and tissues are not meant to live forever as they also have vital parts that wear out with continued use.

Rate of living theory: Based on this theory, the rate of an organism's metabolism determines lifespan, with a faster metabolism resulting in a shorter lifespan.

Cross-linking theory: According to this theory, aging occurs as cross-linked proteins accumulate and damage cells and tissues.

Free-radical theory: This theory proposes that aging is caused by environmental free-radical exposure, which damages DNA, proteins, and lipids. Environmental exposures to cigarette smoke, pollution, and ultraviolet rays contribute to free radical production.

Genome instability theory: This theory states that aging results from damaged DNA, particularly mitochondrial DNA, that the body has been unable to repair. Over time, this damaged DNA accumulates and further hinders the DNA repair process.

Information theory First proposed by Dr. David Sinclair in his book, Lifespan: Why We Age and Why We Don't Have To, this theory attributes aging to a loss of information. As cells become damaged they lose the information encoding their identity. As damage accumulates, more cells lose their identity, and tissue and organ function begins to decline and result in aging.

Can you prevent aging?

What to know about anti-aging habits

As research evolves, aging experts are reframing the aging process. Rather than just a set of innate biological processes that result in irreversible molecular and cellular changes, aging is a complex interaction between genetics and lifestyle. Though you can't fully prevent all aging processes from occurring, research shows that individuals have the power to extend their lifespan by altering key lifestyle aspects like diet, exercise, stress, and sleep.

Science-backed habits to live longer

While longevity may be the ultimate goal, these interventions not only focus on extending lifespan but extending healthspan—the number of years we live in good health—as well.

Eat broccoli sprouts: Broccoli sprouts are packed with sulforaphane, a powerful sulfur-containing compound. Sulforaphane activates pathways in the body that suppress inflammation, activate detoxification, and promote antioxidant action.

Get quality sleep—but not too much: The body's repair mechanisms occur while we sleep. One study examining the sleep habits of 1.3 million individuals found that those who slept between six to nine hours per night had the lowest risk of all-cause mortality compared to those who slept for less than six or more than nine hours per night.

Reduce red meat intake: Red and processed meat intake is associated with a greater risk of all-cause mortality and mortality from cardiovascular disease, the number one cause of death in the United States. According to one study, swapping red meat for plant-based protein sources like beans or tofu is associated with a 13% lower risk of mortality in men and a 15% lower risk of mortality in women.

Consider intermittent fasting: Intermittent fasting contributes to longevity by eliciting the adaptive stress response within the body – a positive type of physiological stress. Adaptive stress activates different pathways in the body that help to increase the production of antioxidants, stimulate DNA repair, decrease inflammation, and clear out dead and damaged cells. [19]

Keep stress levels in check: It is well established that high stress levels negatively impact almost every aspect of health, including longevity. Research shows that those who can manage stress and experience positive emotions like happiness and joy live longer, healthier lives.

Key takeaways

Aging is a decrease in functional capacity over time due to accumulated cellular damage.

There is not one singular explanation as to why we age. Rather, aging is the result of complex interactions between our genetics and our environment.

There are two main categories of aging: programmed theories and damage theories.

Based on the most recent scientific advances, researchers believe that the aging process can be slowed down.

Eating a well-balanced diet, getting enough sleep, and managing stress levels are three key interventions that longevity experts agree on.

In this chapter, we've delved into the intricate and fascinating world of the biology of aging. From cellular senescence to the profound impact of DNA damage, oxidative stress, and hormonal shifts, we've explored the biological underpinnings that shape the path of aging. The interplay of genes, epigenetics, and telomeres has been unveiled, offering insights into the intricate mechanisms that govern our journey through time.

The biology of aging Is a tapestry of complex processes, each thread revealing a deeper understanding of how our bodies evolve over the years. We've explored how our cells age, the role of inflammation in the aging process, and how the immune system adapts with time.

As we conclude this chapter, we stand at the crossroads of knowledge and possibility. Armed with the insights we've gained into the biological foundations of aging, we're poised to take the next steps in our quest for a longer, healthier, and more joyful life. The science of aging is not just an academic endeavor; it's a path toward practical solutions and interventions that can empower us to age with grace, resilience, and vitality.

Our journey continues, and in the chapters to come, we'll explore strategies, innovations, and the latest breakthroughs that bring us closer to the goal of extending our health span and embracing the full potential of our lives. The biology of aging is the foundation upon which we build our understanding, and it sets the stage for the practical wisdom that lies ahead.

Chapter 4
Healthy Eating Habits

In the quest for a longer, healthier, and more joyful life, our journey now leads us to the heart of well-being—nutrition. Welcome to Chapter 4, where we explore "Healthy Eating Habits: Nutrition as the Foundation for Longevity."

As we traverse the landscape of longevity, we find that our daily choices, especially those concerning what we eat, play an integral role in shaping our health and vitality. Nutrition is not just about satisfying hunger; it's about fueling our bodies, fortifying our defenses, and nurturing our potential for enduring well-being.

This chapter is a culinary odyssey, a voyage through the world of wholesome foods, balanced diets, and the science of nutrition. It is here that we discover the profound impact of our dietary choices on the aging process, the prevention of age-related diseases, and the enhancement of our overall quality of life.

We'll explore the principles of a longevity-focused diet, dissecting the benefits of antioxidant-rich foods, and uncovering the significance of macronutrients, micronutrients, and hydration. From the Mediterranean diet to plant-based nutrition, we will journey through the diverse landscapes of dietary wisdom.

Healthy eating habits are not just a recommendation; they are the cornerstone of longevity and vitality. Join us in this chapter as we savor the knowledge, insights, and practical wisdom that nutrition brings to the table. Together, we'll uncover the ingredients for a life well-lived and embark on a culinary adventure That nourishes not just our bodies but our spirits as well.

Researchers analyzed hundreds of studies to identify a diet that optimizes human health and longevity.

They found that diets low in animal protein and high in complex carbohydrates that include periods of fasting are most beneficial for long-term health and life span.

However, the researchers note that their findings simply provide a foundation for understanding and that, in practice, diets should be tailored to individual needs and circumstances.

In around 440 B.C., the Greek physician Hippocrates said "Let food be thy medicine and let thy medicine be food."

Although treating food as medicine is a highly debated concept, many recent studies have demonstrated the wisdom in this statement and how monitoring food quantity Source, type, and timing are crucial for good health.

However, what precisely makes up the optimal diet remains controversial. Growing evidence suggests optimal diets may depend on an interplay of health factors, including age, sex, and genetics.

Recently, researchers reviewed hundreds of nutrition studies from cellular to epidemiological perspectives to identify a "common denominator nutrition pattern" for healthy longevity.

They found that diets including mid-to-high levels of unrefined carbohydrates, a low but sufficient plant-based protein intake, and regular fish consumption were linked to an extended lifespan and healthspan.

A professor of gerontology and biological sciences

"First, diet here is intended as a nutritional lifestyle and not as a 'weight-loss strategy' although maintaining a healthy weight is key. All aspects of the diet are linked to long-term health and longevity."

"Generally when one thinks of a longevity diet, the first thing that comes to mind is what we can add to our diet to live longer. This article is important to raise the awareness that the most striking benefits from studies across species have come from limiting the diet or fasting."

The foundation of the longevity diet

For the study, the researchers analyzed hundreds of studies examining nutrition and delayed aging in short-lived species, nutrient response pathways, caloric restriction, fasting, and diets with various macronutrient and composition levels, such as the keto diet.

The studies analyzed nutrition and diet from multiple angles, from cellular and animal studies to clinical and epidemiological research investigating the lifestyles of centenarians.

In the end, the researchers found that the 'longevity diet' includes:

A legume and whole grain-rich pescatarian or vegetarian diet

30% of calories from vegetable fats such as nuts and olive oil

A low but sufficient protein diet until age 65 and then moderate protein intake

Low sugar and refined carbs

No red or processed meat

Limited white meat

12 hours of eating and 12 of fasting per day

Around three cycles of a five-day fasting-mimicking diet per year

The researchers further noted that, rather than targeting a certain number of calories, diets should aim to keep BMI under 25 and maintain ideal sex and age-specific body fat and lean body mass levels.

Moreover, they wrote that diets should be adapted to individual needs—especially for those over 65—to avoid malnourishment. Those over 65, for example, may become frail from a low-protein diet.

For those without insulin resistance or obesity, high consumption of complex carbohydrates could reduce frailty in this age group and others, the researchers wrote, as it provides energy without increasing insulin and activating glucose signaling pathways.

The researchers also found that periodic fasting between the ages of 18 and 70 could reverse insulin resistance generated by a high-calorie diet and regulate blood pressure, total cholesterol, and inflammation.

A recent study supports these findings. It found that changing from the typical Western diet to one rich in legumes, whole grains, and nuts with reduced red and processed meats is linked to an 8-year-longer life expectancy if started at age 60.

Underlying mechanisms

The researchers noted that diets involving calorie and protein restriction were consistently beneficial, whether in short-lived species or om epidemiological studies and large clinical trials.

They further noted that low but sufficient protein, or a recommended protein intake with high levels of legume consumption, could increase the health span by reducing the intake of amino acids including methionine. Methionine has been linked to increased activity in various pro-aging cellular pathways.

When asked how the longevity diet may benefit health from a clinical perspective, Kristin Kirkpatrick, a registered dietitian nutritionist at the Cleveland Clinic and advisor to Dr. Longo's firm, Prolon, told MNT:

"The diet is primarily plant-based which, based on other similar studies, may contribute to lower risk of chronic conditions such as type 2 diabetes and cardiovascular disease."

"Plant-based diets have also been associated with lower inflammation levels in multiple studies. As inflammation is the base of many diseases, this may contribute to the longevity factors as well," she explained.

The researchers conclude that their findings provide solid foundations for future research into nutritional recommendations for healthy longevity.

When asked about the study's limitations, They stressed that there is no 'one-size-fits-all' approach. The optimal diet, they say, may differ due to factors including sex, age, genetic makeup, and any sensitivities and intolerances, such as an intolerance to gluten.

They recommends people visit A dietician should be consulted before starting a new diet. The patients seek her guidance for sustainable dietary changes .A dietician should be consulted before starting a new diet. The patients seek her guidance for sustainable dietary changes. A dietician should be consulted before starting a new diet. The patients seek her guidance for sustainable dietary changes A dietician should be consulted before starting a new diet. The patients seek her guidance for sustainable dietary changes. A dietician should be consulted before starting a new diet. The patients seek her guidance for sustainable dietary changes. A dietician should be consulted before starting a new diet. The patients seek her guidance for sustainable dietary changes. A dietician should be consulted before starting a new diet. The patients seek her guidance for sustainable dietary changes. A dietician should be consulted before starting a new diet. The patients seek her guidance for sustainable dietary changes. A dietician should be consulted before starting a new diet. The patients seek her guidance for sustainable dietary changes. A dietician should be consulted before starting a new diet. The Patients seek her guidance for sustainable dietary changes. A dietician should be consulted before starting a new diet. The patients seek her guidance for sustainable dietary changes. A dietician should be consulted before starting a new diet. The patients seek her guidance for sustainable dietary changes. A dietician should be consulted before starting a new diet. The patients seek her guidance for sustainable dietary changes A dietician should be consulted before starting a new diet. Kirkpatrick's patients seek her guidance for sustainable dietary changes. should be consulted before starting a new diet. The patients seek her guidance for sustainable dietary changes. A dietician should be consulted before starting a new diet. The patients seek her guidance for sustainable dietary changes A dietician should be consulted before starting a new diet. The patients seek her guidance for sustainable dietary changes.

Chapter Five
The Power of Physical Exercise.

In a world where the rhythm of life often seems to speed up, where schedules grow more crowded and the demands on our time and energy ever-increasing, it's easy to overlook one of the most powerful tools we have at our disposal: physical activity. This chapter, "The Power of Physical Activity," is a celebration of movement, the profound impact it can have on our lives, and the remarkable role it plays in our journey toward a long and joyful existence. Physical activity isn't just about exercise; it's about embracing the simple act of moving, whether it's a stroll through a park, a vigorous dance in the living room, or a committed fitness routine at the gym. In these pages, we will dive deep into the science behind it, exploring how exercise affects not only our bodies but also our minds. We will learn how it combats the aging process, fortifies our defenses against disease, and infuses our lives with boundless energy. This chapter is your guide to understanding how physical activity isn't a mere habit; it's a lifeline to a better, healthier, and more vibrant future. It's about discovering a newfound zest for life and, more importantly, sustaining it. Let's lace up our sneakers, roll out the yoga mat, or simply start with a few gentle stretches. Together, we'll unlock the potential of physical activity on our path to a long and joyful life.

Exercise and other daily physical Activities can greatly help make you stay healthier and protect your body from the occurrence of some health disorders. Some of the powers of Physical Activities include ;
Physical Health Benefits: Exercise is essential for maintaining a healthy body. It improves cardiovascular health, strengthens muscles and bones, and helps with weight management. These benefits can extend your lifespan and reduce the risk of chronic diseases. Mental Well-being: Regular exercise has a profound impact on mental health. It releases endorphins, which can reduce stress, anxiety, and depression. Exercise is often prescribed as a complementary therapy for mental health disorders. Cognitive Function: Physical activity can enhance cognitive function and boost creativity. It improves blood flow to the brain, which can enhance memory, focus, and problem-solving abilities. Productivity and Energy: Engaging in regular exercise can increase overall energy levels and productivity. It

can help you stay alert and maintain high energy throughout the day. Lifestyle and Habit Formation: Encouraging regular exercise can lead to positive lifestyle changes. It promotes discipline, time management, and the development of healthy habits. Community and Social Aspects: Exercise can be a social activity, fostering connections with others who share similar fitness goals. These social bonds can be a source of motivation and support. Self-esteem and Body Image: Achieving fitness goals can boost self-esteem and promote a positive body image. This can lead to greater self-confidence and self-acceptance. Longevity: Exercise can potentially extend one's lifespan by reducing the risk of various diseases and promoting overall health and well-being.

Engaging in various types of physical activities can significantly reduce the risk of numerous health disorders. Here are some examples of physical activities and the health benefits associated with them:

1. Aerobic Exercise (e.g., Running, Cycling, Swimming): Aerobic activities improve cardiovascular health, reduce the risk of heart disease, lower blood pressure, and help manage weight. They also boost mood and reduce the risk of depression.

2. Strength Training (e.g., Weightlifting, Resistance Exercises): Strength training increases muscle mass, bone density, and metabolism. It can reduce the risk of osteoporosis, improve insulin sensitivity, and enhance overall physical performance.

3. Yoga: Yoga promotes flexibility, balance, and relaxation. It can alleviate stress, improve mental well-being, and reduce the risk of chronic conditions such as hypertension and arthritis.

4. Pilates: Pilates focuses on core strength and flexibility. It can improve posture, reduce the risk of back pain, and enhance overall body awareness.

5. Tai Chi: Tai Chi combines gentle movements with mindfulness. It can improve balance, reduce the risk of falls in older adults, and may lower blood pressure.

6. Dancing: Dancing not only provides physical exercise but also fosters social interaction and coordination. It can be an enjoyable way to reduce the risk of cardiovascular disease and improve mental health.

7. Hiking and Nature Walks: These activities promote both physical and mental well-being. They reduce stress, encourage physical fitness, and can be a part of a healthy lifestyle.

8. Swimming: Swimming is a low-impact exercise that is easy on the joints. It can improve cardiovascular fitness, lung capacity, and overall muscle tone.

9. Cycling: Biking is a great way to build leg strength and improve cardiovascular health. It's also an eco-friendly mode of transportation.

10. Martial Arts (e.g., Karate, Judo): Martial arts enhance physical fitness, flexibility, and self-defense skills. They promote discipline and self-confidence.

By incorporating a variety of these activities into your routine, you can reduce the risk of health disorders such as heart disease, obesity, diabetes, osteoporosis, and mental health issues. The key is to find activities that you enjoy and can sustain in the long term, making physical fitness an integral part of your lifestyle.

In conclusion, the power of physical exercise is undeniable and far-reaching. It transcends mere physical fitness, touching every facet of our lives. From enhancing our physical health and mental well-being to fostering discipline, social connections, and self-esteem, exercise is a holistic tool for self-improvement.

Through exercise, we not only strengthen our bodies but also fortify our minds, creating a synergy that empowers us to tackle life's challenges with resilience and vigor. The journey of adopting a regular exercise routine is a path to self-discovery, personal growth, and a longer, healthier life.

As you reflect on the insights shared in this chapter, may you find inspiration to embark on your fitness journey or encourage others to harness the transformative potential of physical exercise? It is a journey worth taking, for it leads not only to a healthier body but to a richer, more fulfilling life.

CHAPTER SIX
The Importance of Quality sleep

In the relentless pursuit of health, happiness, and longevity, there's a profound but often overlooked aspect of our lives that holds the key to all three: quality sleep. Welcome to a chapter dedicated to unraveling the significance of slumber, to understand how the hours we spend in repose shape not only our dreams but our waking lives as well. Sleep is far more than the mere absence of wakefulness; it's a realm where our bodies heal, our minds rejuvenate, and our spirits find solace. In these pages, we venture into the realm of dreams and deep rest, exploring the critical role sleep plays in our well-being. We'll uncover the science of sleep, the mysteries of its stages, and the profound impact it has on our physical and mental health. This chapter is a journey into the quiet hours of the night, the place where our bodies recharge and our souls find peace. As we delve into the importance of quality sleep, we'll unearth practical insights, strategies, and wisdom to enhance our nightly repose. Join us in this exploration of the secrets hidden within the world of slumber, for they hold the power to extend our years and make them profoundly more joyful. Here, we embark on a voyage through the lands of dreams, deep slumbers, and the secrets that lie within. So, let's begin the journey into the heart of the night, where the true fountain of youth may very well be found.

Quality sleep is the unsung hero of health and well-being, a vital cornerstone on which our physical, mental, and emotional health is built. In your book, it's essential to emphasize the paramount importance of quality sleep in the quest for a long and joyful life. Here are some key points to consider when explaining its importance:

1. Physical Restoration: Quality sleep is the time when our bodies engage in profound repair and renewal. During deep slumber, tissues are repaired, muscles rebuilt, and the immune system recharges. This is crucial for maintaining overall health, vitality, and longevity.

2. Cognitive Function: Sleep is the brain's time to tidy up and process information. Adequate, quality sleep is vital for memory consolidation, problem-solving,

creativity, and overall cognitive function. It enables us to think, make better decisions, and adapt to new challenges.

3. Emotional Well-Being: A lack of sleep can lead to mood swings, irritability, and increased stress levels. Quality sleep contributes to emotional stability and resilience, enhancing our ability to handle life's ups and downs with grace.

4. Hormone Regulation: Sleep plays a pivotal role in regulating hormones, including cortisol and melatonin. A disrupted sleep pattern can lead to imbalances in these hormones, which are linked to stress, weight management, and overall health.

5. Immune Function: The immune system is bolstered during sleep, enhancing our ability to fend off illnesses and infections. Inadequate sleep weakens our immune defenses, making us more susceptible to disease.

6. Heart Health: Quality sleep supports cardiovascular health by reducing the risk of hypertension and heart disease. It aids in maintaining healthy blood pressure and heart rate.

7. Longevity: Numerous studies have shown that people who consistently get quality sleep tend to live longer, healthier lives. Sleep contributes to our body's natural ability to repair itself, slowing the aging process.

8. Stress Management: Quality sleep is a natural stress reducer. It equips us with the mental and emotional resilience to face stressors more effectively.

9. Weight Management: Sleep is intricately connected to our body's regulation of appetite and metabolism. Poor sleep patterns can lead to weight gain, making quality sleep an essential component of a healthy lifestyle.

10. Preventing Chronic Diseases: Chronic sleep deprivation has been linked to a higher risk of developing chronic diseases, including diabetes, obesity, and certain cancers. Ensuring quality sleep is a preventive measure against these conditions.

Quality sleep isn't a luxury but a fundamental requirement for overall health and longevity. It's the secret ingredient to a longer, more joyful life, enabling us to be our best selves, both physically and mentally.

Science of sleep:

Sleep is a complex and fascinating phenomenon that has intrigued scientists and researchers for many years. It's not merely a passive state of rest; instead, it's a highly active and regulated process that consists of several distinct stages. Understanding the science of sleep involves exploring the physiological and neurological mechanisms that govern this essential aspect of our lives.

Sleep Stages:
Sleep is typically divided into two main categories: rapid-eye movement (REM) sleep and non-rapid-eye movement (NREM) sleep.

1. NREM Sleep: This stage is further divided into three sub-stages: N1, N2, and N3.

   - N1 (NREM Stage 1): The transition from wakefulness to sleep. It's a light stage where you can be easily awakened. Muscle activity decreases, and your eye movements are slow.

   - N2 (NREM Stage 2): A deeper stage where heart rate and body temperature decrease. Sleep spindles (short bursts of brain activity) and K-complexes (sharp, high-voltage brain waves) are commonly seen.

   - N3 (NREM Stage 3): Also known as slow-wave sleep, it's the deepest and most restorative stage. During N3, the body undergoes essential repair and maintenance. It's challenging to wake someone in this stage, and it's when growth hormone is released.

2. REM Sleep: Rapid eye movement sleep is the stage associated with vivid dreaming. It's characterized by increased brain activity, rapid eye movements, and temporary paralysis of major muscle groups. Despite the heightened brain activity, the body is effectively immobilized to prevent acting out dreams.

Circadian Rhythms:
Our sleep-wake cycle is governed by circadian rhythms, which are roughly 24-hour cycles influenced by external cues like light and temperature. The suprachiasmatic nucleus (SCN) in the brain's hypothalamus acts as our internal clock. It regulates the release of melatonin, a hormone that makes us feel drowsy in the evening and wakeful in the morning.

Homeostasis:
Sleep pressure, or the drive to sleep, accumulates as we stay awake. Adenosine, a neurotransmitter, builds up in the brain throughout the day and promotes sleep when its levels are high. Sleep helps to clear adenosine, reducing our need for sleep.

Sleep Disorders:
Disruptions in the sleep process can lead to sleep disorders, including insomnia, sleep apnea, restless legs syndrome, narcolepsy, and parasomnias like sleepwalking. These conditions result from imbalances in sleep stages, neurotransmitter function, or circadian rhythms.

Understanding the science of sleep helps us appreciate the complexity of this fundamental biological process. It also underscores the importance of achieving a balanced and restful sleep pattern, as disturbances in the science of sleep can have profound effects on physical and mental health, productivity, and overall well-being.

BENEFITS OF QUALITY SLEEP

1. Enhanced Immune Function: Quality sleep is like a boost for your immune system. During restorative sleep, your body produces and releases cytokines, a type of protein that helps fight infection, inflammation, and stress. A lack of quality sleep can weaken your immune defenses, making you more susceptible to illnesses and infections.

2. Improved Cardiovascular Health: Consistent, good-quality sleep supports heart health. It helps regulate blood pressure, reduces stress on the cardiovascular system, and decreases the risk of heart disease. Over time, inadequate sleep may contribute to conditions like hypertension, which can lead to more severe cardiovascular issues.

3. Hormone Regulation: Sleep is intricately linked to hormone regulation. Two hormones, in particular, are affected by sleep quality: melatonin and cortisol. Melatonin, which is produced during the night, helps regulate your sleep-wake cycle. Cortisol, often referred to as the stress hormone, is also influenced by sleep patterns. Disruptions in these hormones due to poor sleep can lead to stress, weight gain, and metabolic imbalances.

4. Cognitive Function: Quality sleep is essential for optimal brain function. During deep sleep, memories are consolidated, and the brain clears out waste products. This enhances cognitive functions such as memory, problem-solving, creativity, and concentration. Good-quality sleep is crucial for mental clarity and productivity.

5. Emotional Well-Being: A lack of quality sleep can lead to mood disturbances, including irritability, anxiety, and depression. Adequate sleep supports emotional stability, helping you manage stress and cope with life's challenges more effectively.

6. Stress Reduction: Quality sleep reduces the production of stress hormones like cortisol. This means you're better equipped to handle stressors in your daily life. It's a natural stress-reduction method that contributes to overall emotional and psychological well-being.

7. Weight Management: Sleep patterns play a significant role in regulating appetite and metabolism. Poor sleep can lead to imbalances in hormones that control hunger and fullness, which can contribute to weight gain. Quality sleep is a valuable component of a healthy lifestyle, particularly when it comes to maintaining a healthy weight.

8. Prevention of Chronic Diseases: Chronic sleep deprivation has been linked to an increased risk of developing chronic health conditions, including diabetes, obesity,

and certain types of cancer. Prioritizing quality sleep can act as a preventive measure against these diseases.

9. Pain Management; Sleep is essential for the body's healing processes. Adequate rest helps manage and reduce pain, especially chronic pain conditions. It can improve pain tolerance and decrease discomfort.

10. Longevity: Numerous studies have shown that individuals who consistently get quality sleep tend to live longer, healthier lives. Sleep's role in bodily repair and slowing the aging process contributes to an increased lifespan.

Incorporating good-quality sleep into your daily routine is a fundamental aspect of maintaining and improving your overall health and well-being. Understanding these health benefits can motivate you to prioritize sleep and reap the rewards of a healthier and more fulfilling life.

Common Sleep Disorders

Some of the common sleep Disorders include ;
1. Insomnia: Insomnia is characterized by difficulty falling asleep, staying asleep, or experiencing non-restorative sleep. It can be acute (short-term) or chronic (long-term). Factors such as stress, anxiety, depression, and poor sleep habits can contribute to insomnia. Treatment may involve behavioral therapy, lifestyle changes, or, in some cases, medications.

2. Sleep Apnea: Sleep apnea is a condition in which breathing repeatedly stops and starts during sleep. There are two main types: obstructive sleep apnea (OSA), caused by a physical obstruction in the airway, and central sleep apnea, which is related to a failure of the brain to signal the muscles to breathe. Sleep apnea can lead to snoring, daytime fatigue, and potentially serious health issues, including heart disease. Treatments include lifestyle changes, continuous positive airway pressure (CPAP) therapy, or in some cases, surgery.

3. Restless Legs Syndrome (RLS): RLS is a neurological disorder characterized by an irresistible urge to move the legs, often due to uncomfortable sensations such as crawling, tingling, or aching. Symptoms usually occur when at rest and worsen in

the evening or at night, which can disrupt sleep. Lifestyle changes and medications can help manage RLS.

4. Narcolepsy: Narcolepsy is a chronic neurological disorder characterized by excessive daytime sleepiness and sudden sleep attacks. People with narcolepsy may experience cataplexy (sudden muscle weakness or paralysis), sleep paralysis, and vivid hallucinations when falling asleep or waking up. Treatment often involves medications to manage symptoms.

5. Parasomnias: Parasomnias are abnormal behaviors that occur during sleep. They can include sleepwalking, night terrors, and sleeptalking. These behaviors can disrupt sleep for both the individual experiencing them and their bed partner. Managing parasomnias often involves improving sleep hygiene and, in some cases, medication.

6. Circadian Rhythm Disorders: Circadian rhythm disorders occur when the body's internal clock is misaligned with the desired sleep-wake schedule. Conditions like jet lag, shift work sleep disorder, and delayed sleep-wake phase disorder can lead to sleep disturbances. Strategies to reset the internal clock may be employed, such as light therapy, melatonin supplements, or adjusting work schedules.

7. Hypersomnia: Hypersomnia is characterized by excessive daytime sleepiness, leading to prolonged and unrefreshing daytime naps. It can result from underlying medical conditions and may require treatment for the primary cause.

8. Sleep-related Movement Disorders: Conditions like periodic limb movement disorder (PLMD) and restless leg syndrome (RLS) involve involuntary movements during sleep that can lead to awakenings and poor sleep quality. Medications and lifestyle adjustments can be used to manage these disorders.

Understanding these common sleep disorders is essential for recognizing their symptoms and seeking appropriate diagnosis and treatment. If you suspect you have a sleep disorder, it's advisable to consult a healthcare professional or sleep specialist for a thorough evaluation and personalized treatment plan.

Stress Reduction techniques

Stress reduction techniques are essential for maintaining mental and emotional well-being. Here are some effective strategies for managing and reducing stress:

1. Deep Breathing and Relaxation Techniques:
   - Deep breathing exercises, such as diaphragmatic breathing, can help calm the nervous system and reduce stress. Incorporate relaxation techniques like progressive muscle relaxation, guided imagery, or meditation to promote a sense of calm and relaxation.

2. Physical Activity:
   - Regular physical activity, such as walking, jogging, yoga, or even dancing, can reduce stress hormones and stimulate the release of endorphins, which are natural mood lifters. Aim for at least 30 minutes of exercise most days of the week.

3. Mindfulness and Meditation:
   - Mindfulness meditation practices encourage living in the present moment and accepting it without judgment. This can help reduce rumination on past or future stressors. Guided mindfulness and meditation apps are widely available to assist in daily practice.

4. Time Management and Organization:
   - Effective time management helps prevent feelings of being overwhelmed and stressed. Use tools like calendars, to-do lists, and prioritization to manage tasks and projects efficiently.

5. Social Support:
   - Talking to friends, family, or a therapist can provide emotional support and perspective. Sharing your feelings and concerns can help relieve stress and provide insight into solutions.

6. Healthy Eating:
   - A well-balanced diet can have a significant impact on stress management. Avoid excessive caffeine and sugar, and opt for nutritious foods rich in vitamins, minerals, and antioxidants.

7. Adequate Sleep:

- Prioritizing good-quality sleep is crucial for stress reduction. Aim for 7-9 hours of sleep each night to help your body recover from daily stressors.

8. Setting Boundaries:
   - Learn to say no to additional commitments or responsibilities when your plate is already full. Setting boundaries is essential for preventing excessive stress.

9. Hobbies and Leisure Activities:
   - Engaging in hobbies and activities you enjoy can provide a break from stressors and promote relaxation. Whether it's reading, art, music, or sports, make time for what brings you joy.

10. Cognitive Behavioral Techniques:
   - Cognitive-behavioral therapy (CBT) is a therapeutic approach that helps individuals identify and change negative thought patterns and behaviors. It can be beneficial for managing stress and anxiety.

11. Nature and Outdoors:
   - Spending time in nature, even a short walk in a park, can reduce stress and improve mental well-being. It's known as "eco-therapy."

12. Gratitude and Journaling:
   - Keeping a gratitude journal and focusing on positive aspects of your life can shift your perspective and reduce stress. Writing down your thoughts and feelings can also provide a healthy emotional outlet.

13. Seek Professional Help:
   - If stress becomes overwhelming and begins to affect your daily life, consider seeking help from a mental health professional. They can provide guidance and therapeutic support tailored to your specific needs.

Remember that stress is a natural part of life, but how you respond to it can greatly impact your well-being. By incorporating these stress reduction techniques into your daily routine, you can build resilience and better manage life's challenges.

Creating the Ideal Sleep Environment

Creating the Ideal Sleep Environment" refers to the practice of setting up your bedroom in a way that promotes and enhances the quality of your sleep. The bedroom is the space where you spend a significant portion of your life, and its surroundings can have a profound impact on your ability to rest, relax, and achieve restorative sleep. Here's an explanation of this concept:

1. Light and Darkness: Ensure that your bedroom is conducive to sleep by keeping it dark when you need to sleep. This may involve using blackout curtains to block out streetlights or early morning sun. Reducing exposure to light in the evening helps your body produce melatonin, a hormone that regulates your sleep-wake cycle.

2. Comfortable Bedding: Invest in a comfortable mattress and pillows that suit your preferences. The right bedding can significantly improve your sleep quality by providing proper support and comfort. Choosing the right bedding materials, such as sheets and blankets, can also help regulate temperature and comfort.

3. Temperature Control: A comfortable bedroom temperature is vital for quality sleep. Most people sleep best in a slightly cool room, usually between 60 to 67 degrees Fahrenheit (15 to 20 degrees Celsius). Adjust your thermostat or use bedding materials like sheets and blankets to maintain an ideal temperature.

4. Minimize Noise: Reducing noise in your sleep environment is crucial for quality rest. Earplugs or white noise machines can help mask disruptive sounds like traffic or noisy neighbors. Alternatively, consider using soft materials such as heavy curtains or carpets to dampen noise.

5. Bedroom Clutter: A clutter-free environment can promote relaxation. Organize your bedroom to minimize distractions and create a calming atmosphere. A tidy, uncluttered space can reduce stress and promote better sleep.

6. Electronic Devices: Minimize the presence of electronic devices in your bedroom, particularly those with bright screens. The blue light emitted from screens can interfere with your body's melatonin production, making it more difficult to fall asleep. Consider creating a screen-free zone in your bedroom.

7. Soothing Colors and Decor: The choice of colors and decor in your bedroom can influence your mood and relaxation. Soft, soothing colors and decor can create a calming atmosphere, helping you wind down before sleep.

8. Air Quality: Ensure good air quality in your bedroom by maintaining proper ventilation. Fresh air and a well-ventilated space can improve your sleep environment. Consider using an air purifier if needed.

9. Personalization: Tailor your sleep environment to your personal preferences. Everyone has unique needs and preferences for their sleep space. Experiment with different elements until you find the combination that best suits your sleep style.

Optimizing your bedroom for quality sleep is a crucial step in achieving restful and restorative nights. By considering and adjusting these various factors in your sleep environment, you can create a space that promotes relaxation, minimizes disturbances, and sets the stage for a better night's sleep.

In the quest for a longer, happier, and healthier life, we have explored various facets of well-being, and one of the most foundational yet often overlooked elements is the quality of our sleep. As we conclude this chapter, it's essential to recognize that our bedroom is the stage upon which the drama of sleep unfolds, and it's within this environment that we have the power to script the ideal setting for a night of truly restorative rest. The secrets to a long and joyful life lie not only in the mysteries of diet and exercise but also in the embrace of tranquility that a well-prepared sleep environment can offer. In these carefully chosen elements — from the gentle play of light and darkness to the comfort of our bedding, the serenity of a clutter-free space, and the soothing decor that surrounds us — we discover the means to not just sleep but to rejuvenate our bodies, minds, and spirits. The American Fountain of You is not a place or a spring, but a lifestyle choice, a commitment to nurturing the many aspects of our well-being, and a recognition that, in the confines of our bedrooms, we hold a powerful tool for achieving the longevity and joy we seek. So, dear readers, as you prepare to rest your heads, remember that your bedroom is more than a room; it's a sanctuary where dreams are born, and where the secrets of a long and joyful life may just be found. Good night, and may your dreams be both peaceful and profound."

Chapter Seven

Cultivating Connections for a Fulfilling Life

In a world that often moves at a frenetic pace, where digital screens and devices dominate our interactions, it's easy to overlook one of the most profound secrets to a long and joyful life: meaningful connections. Chapter Eight of our journey delves into the pivotal role that relationships play in nurturing our well-being, enhancing our longevity, and providing a profound sense of fulfillment. We are inherently social creatures, wired for connection, empathy, and companionship. The bonds we forge with family, friends, and communities serve as the invisible threads that weave the tapestry of a rich and purposeful existence. In this chapter, we embark on a deep exploration of the science and art of cultivating these connections, for they are a source of nourishment for the soul, capable of transforming our lives in countless ways. From the power of human touch to the art of active listening, we'll uncover the mysteries of what makes relationships flourish. We'll explore the profound physical and psychological benefits of robust social connections, and we'll unlock the secrets to building and maintaining them. The joy and longevity of your life might very well be interwoven with the quality of your connections, and this chapter is your guide to cultivating those bonds for a life that is not just long but extraordinarily joyful.

The science of connection explores the profound and multifaceted impact that social connections and relationships have on our physical, mental, and emotional well-being. This field of study delves into the physiological and psychological mechanisms that underlie our need for social bonds and the far-reaching effects they have on our lives. Here's an explanation of the science of connection:

1. Hormonal and Neurological Responses: Social connections trigger the release of hormones and neurotransmitters that influence our feelings and behaviors. For example, when we bond with others, our bodies release oxytocin, often referred to as the "love hormone." Oxytocin promotes bonding, trust, and social attachment. In contrast, stress hormones like cortisol decrease in the presence of strong social support.

2. Immune System Function: Strong social connections can bolster the immune system. People with robust social networks tend to have better immune function, making them more resilient against infections and diseases.

3. Pain Regulation: The brain's response to pain can be influenced by social connections. Touch and social interaction trigger the release of endorphins, natural painkillers that reduce discomfort.

4. Stress Reduction: Social support and connections are crucial for stress reduction. Close relationships provide emotional support and coping mechanisms, helping individuals manage stress more effectively. Studies have shown that people with strong social connections tend to experience less stress and have better mental health.

5. Mental Health: Loneliness and social isolation are associated with an increased risk of mental health conditions, including depression and anxiety. In contrast, positive social interactions and relationships can enhance mental well-being and promote resilience in the face of life's challenges.

6. Longevity: Numerous studies have shown that individuals with strong social connections tend to live longer, healthier lives. Social support can be a protective factor against mortality, particularly in older adults.

7. Cognitive Function: Engagement in social activities and meaningful conversations can enhance cognitive function and protect against cognitive decline. Staying socially active is associated with improved memory, problem-solving, and overall mental acuity.

8. Empathy and Altruism: Our ability to connect with others is linked to our capacity for empathy and altruism. Empathy allows us to understand and relate to the emotions of others, promoting a sense of compassion and unity.

9. Human Evolution: The need for social connections is deeply rooted in our evolutionary history. Humans are social animals, and our survival and success as a species have depended on our ability to cooperate, form bonds, and work together in groups.

10. Psychological Resilience: Strong social connections are linked to psychological resilience. People with a robust support network tend to recover more quickly from challenging life events and adapt more effectively to change.

The science of connection highlights the essential role of relationships in our lives. It demonstrates that humans are wired for social interactions, and our well-being is deeply intertwined with the quality of our connections. This understanding underscores the importance of nurturing and maintaining meaningful relationships to promote physical health, mental well-being, and emotional fulfillment.

LONGEVITY IN BLUE ZONES

Blue Zones are regions in the world known for having exceptionally high concentrations of centenarians, people who live to be 100 years old or more. These regions have attracted the attention of researchers and health experts due to their remarkable longevity and lower rates of age-related diseases. There are several Blue Zones worldwide, and they offer insights into the factors that contribute to long and healthy lives. Some well-known Blue Zones include:

1. Okinawa, Japan: Okinawa is famous for having one of the world's highest life expectancies. The Okinawan diet, which is rich in vegetables, tofu, and fish, is often credited for their longevity. Additionally, a strong sense of community and purpose in life plays a crucial role in the health and well-being of Okinawans.

2. Sardinia, Italy: Sardinia's mountainous regions are home to a large number of centenarians. The Sardinian diet, rich in whole grains, legumes, and goat's milk, is thought to be a contributing factor. Strong family and community bonds are also integral to their long and healthy lives.

3. Nicoya Peninsula, Costa Rica: The Nicoyan diet, which includes beans, corn, and tropical fruits, is believed to promote longevity. Active lifestyles, a sense of community, and a strong family structure contribute to their exceptional life expectancy.

4. Ikaria, Greece: Ikaria, known as the "island where people forget to die," is characterized by a Mediterranean diet, rich in olive oil, vegetables, and herbs.

Daily physical activity, strong social connections, and a relaxed lifestyle are central to the health and longevity of its residents.

5. Loma Linda, California, USA: Loma Linda is a Blue Zone in the United States, and it is primarily home to a community of Seventh-day Adventists. Their vegetarian diet, regular exercise, and strong faith-based connections are contributing factors to their longevity.

Key factors that are often associated with Blue Zones and their residents' longevity include:

- Diet: Blue Zone diets typically emphasize plant-based foods, whole grains, legumes, and healthy fats like olive oil. These diets are low in processed foods, sugar, and red meat.

- Physical Activity: Blue Zone communities engage in regular physical activity as part of their daily lives. This may involve gardening, walking, or other forms of low-intensity exercise.

- Strong Social Connections: Close-knit communities, family bonds, and social engagement are common features of Blue Zones. These connections provide emotional support and a sense of purpose.

- Stress Reduction: Blue Zone residents often have low-stress lifestyles, which can contribute to better health and longevity.

- Purpose in Life: Having a sense of purpose and meaning in life is associated with better mental and physical health in Blue Zones.

These regions offer valuable insights into the factors that can promote longevity and a high quality of life. While genetics play a role, lifestyle, and environment also have a significant impact on health and longevity. Researchers continue to study Blue Zones to better understand how to apply these principles in other parts of the world to improve overall well-being.

The Power of Community

In the grand tapestry of life, there exists a profound secret to a long and joyful existence, one that we often overlook in our fast-paced, modern world — the power of community. This chapter takes us on a journey to uncover the transformative force that communities offer, not merely as a collection of individuals but as a source of nourishment for the human spirit. Community represents the shared bonds, values, and aspirations that unite people, creating a sense of belonging and purpose. It is a force that transcends individuals and shapes cultures, societies, and lifespans. The power of community goes beyond social gatherings; it touches upon the very essence of human connection, empathy, and collaboration. As we delve into this chapter, we'll explore how communities can impact well-being and longevity. We'll dissect the science of social support, the psychological benefits of belonging, and the remarkable stories of individuals whose lives have been enriched and extended by their bonds with others. The pursuit of a long and joyful life isn't merely an individual endeavor; it is profoundly intertwined with the communities we create and the networks we nurture.

Relationships and stress are closely intertwined, and the nature of our connections with others can significantly impact our stress levels. Here's an explanation of the relationship between relationships and stress:

The Impact of Relationships on Stress:

1. Social Support: Positive, supportive relationships can act as a buffer against stress. When we have a strong support network of friends, family, and loved ones, we often feel more resilient in the face of life's challenges. Knowing that you have people who care about your well-being and are there to lend a listening ear or offer assistance can reduce the perception of stress.

2. Emotional Regulation: Sharing your feelings and experiences with someone you trust can help you process emotions and alleviate stress. When you can express your worries, fears, or frustrations to a supportive person, it can provide emotional relief and reduce the burden of stress.

3. Sense of Belonging: Feeling connected to a community or social group fosters a sense of belonging. This feeling of inclusion can reduce stress, as it provides a psychological safety net, particularly in times of difficulty.

4. Conflict and Strain: On the flip side, strained or conflict-ridden relationships can contribute to stress. Discord within relationships, whether in a marriage, family or at work, can create ongoing stressors that affect mental and emotional well-being.

5. Caregiver Stress: Providing care for a loved one who is ill or in need can be emotionally taxing, leading to caregiver stress. This form of stress can affect family relationships, especially if there's a lack of support from others.

6. Interpersonal Conflict at Work: Workplace relationships and interactions with colleagues and supervisors can be significant sources of stress. A hostile work environment, conflicts with coworkers, or demanding bosses can contribute to job-related stress.

7. Loneliness and Isolation: Loneliness and social isolation can lead to stress and mental health issues. A lack of meaningful connections can leave individuals feeling isolated, contributing to stress and anxiety.

Managing Relationship-Related Stress:

1. Effective Communication: Open and honest communication is key to resolving conflicts and misunderstandings within relationships. Addressing issues constructively can reduce stress and improve the quality of the relationship.

2. Setting Boundaries: Establishing and maintaining healthy boundaries within relationships can help prevent excessive stress. Knowing when to say no or take a step back when needed is crucial for managing stress.

3. Conflict Resolution Skills: Developing effective conflict resolution skills can help navigate and resolve disputes within relationships, reducing ongoing sources of stress.

4. Seeking Support: When relationship-related stress becomes overwhelming, seeking support from a therapist or counselor can be beneficial. They can guide managing stress and improving relationship dynamics.

5. Balancing Personal Time: Taking time for self-care and relaxation is essential for managing stress in any relationship. It allows individuals to recharge and maintain their well-being.

Understanding the complex relationship between social connections and stress is crucial for maintaining healthy relationships and managing stress effectively. Positive relationships can act as a powerful antidote to stress, while strained relationships can contribute to its onset. By nurturing supportive connections and developing effective coping strategies, individuals can create a healthier, less stressful social environment.

Act with kindness and empathy.
Acts of kindness and empathy are powerful human behaviors that foster positive interactions, strengthen relationships, and contribute to the well-being of individuals and communities. Here's an explanation of these two concepts:

Acts of Kindness:
Acts of kindness refer to intentional, selfless actions that are aimed at benefiting others. These actions can be small, such as holding the door for someone, or more significant, like volunteering at a local charity. The essence of kindness lies in the genuine desire to make another person's life better without expecting anything in return.

- Positive Impact: Acts of kindness have a positive impact on both the giver and the recipient. They can brighten someone's day, alleviate stress, and create a sense of connection and goodwill.

- Boosting Well-Being: Engaging in acts of kindness can boost the giver's mood and overall well-being. It triggers the release of "feel-good" hormones, such as oxytocin and endorphins, which contribute to a sense of happiness and contentment.

- Strengthening Relationships: Kindness is a foundation for building and maintaining strong, healthy relationships. Small acts of kindness within a relationship can strengthen bonds and create trust.

- Creating a Positive Ripple Effect: Acts of kindness can set in motion a ripple effect, inspiring others to be kind as well. This creates a more compassionate and supportive community.

Empathy:
Empathy is the ability to understand and share the feelings and perspectives of another person. It involves not just recognizing someone else's emotions but also connecting with and feeling them on some level. Empathy is crucial for meaningful and compassionate interactions with others.

- Emotional Connection: Empathy allows people to establish emotional connections and deepen their relationships. When someone feels understood and validated, it fosters a sense of trust and intimacy.

- Conflict Resolution: In conflicts or disagreements, empathy can help bridge differences by enabling individuals to see the situation from another's viewpoint. This understanding can lead to more constructive resolutions.

- Enhanced Communication: Empathetic communication involves active listening, asking open-ended questions, and validating the other person's feelings. This type of communication fosters understanding and supportive relationships.

- Reducing Prejudice: Empathy can help break down stereotypes and prejudices by allowing individuals to see beyond their biases and understand the experiences of people from diverse backgrounds.

- Building a Caring Society: A society that values and promotes empathy is more likely to address social issues, support those in need, and create a sense of collective responsibility.

Both acts of kindness and empathy contribute to a more compassionate and interconnected world. Acts of kindness are tangible actions that demonstrate empathy, and empathy is the emotional foundation that allows us to engage in acts of kindness. By practicing these behaviors, we create a more empathetic, caring, and supportive community and foster personal well-being and positive relationships.

Friendship plays a significant and multifaceted role in our lives, contributing to our well-being, happiness, and overall quality of life. Here's an explanation of the role of friendship:

The Role of Friendship:

1. Emotional Support: Friends provide a vital source of emotional support. They are there to listen, offer empathy, and provide comfort during challenging times. Sharing your joys and sorrows with friends can be a cathartic and emotionally uplifting experience.

2. Social Connection: Friendship fosters a sense of social connection and belonging. It counters feelings of loneliness and isolation by providing a network of people who understand, care about, and value your company.

3. Shared Experiences: Friends are companions in the journey of life. They share experiences, memories, and adventures, making life more meaningful and enjoyable. The shared history and inside jokes create a unique bond.

4. Stress Reduction: Quality friendships can help reduce stress. Spending time with friends, and engaging in laughter and enjoyable activities, can lead to the release of endorphins, which are natural mood lifters and stress reducers.

5. Enhanced Well-Being: Research has shown that people with strong social connections, including friendships, tend to have better mental health and physical well-being. Friendships contribute to overall life satisfaction and happiness.

6. Confidants: Friends often serve as trusted confidants with whom you can discuss personal matters, seek advice, and receive honest feedback. This safe space for sharing thoughts and feelings is essential for personal growth.

7. Support System: Friends provide a support system in times of crisis, whether it's illness, loss, or personal setbacks. They offer practical assistance, emotional comfort, and a sense of security.

8. Companionship: Friends are companions for various activities and hobbies. They encourage and motivate us to try new things, pursue interests, and lead a more enriched life.

9. Diverse Perspectives: Friendships expose us to diverse viewpoints and backgrounds. They challenge our beliefs and broaden our horizons, fostering personal growth and tolerance.

10. Longevity: Research suggests that individuals with strong social connections, including friendships, tend to live longer and have a lower risk of various health conditions. Friends provide a sense of purpose and motivation to stay active and engaged.

11. Quality Over Quantity: The quality of friendships is more important than the quantity. Meaningful, authentic friendships are often more fulfilling than a large number of acquaintances.

12. Reciprocity and Trust: Friendship is built on trust, reciprocity, and mutual support. Friends are reliable and trustworthy, and these qualities underpin the strength of the relationship.

Friendship enriches our lives in countless ways, providing emotional support, camaraderie, and a sense of connection. It plays a pivotal role in our mental and physical well-being, contributing to a longer, happier, and more fulfilling life. Cultivating and nurturing friendships is a lifelong endeavor that brings with it a host of benefits and rewards.

Virtual and physical connections
Virtual and physical connections represent two distinct modes of interaction and relationship-building in the digital age. Each offers its own set of advantages and challenges. Here's an explanation of both:

Virtual Connections:

1. Online Social Networks: Virtual connections are often established through online social networks such as Facebook, Twitter, and Instagram. These platforms

enable individuals to connect with people around the world, share information, and engage in conversations.

2. Global Reach: Virtual connections have the advantage of a global reach. You can connect with individuals from different cultures and backgrounds, broadening your perspectives and experiences.

3. Convenience: Virtual connections are convenient. You can interact with others from the comfort of your home or anywhere with an internet connection, making it accessible and flexible.

4. Information Sharing: Virtual connections facilitate the sharing of information, news, and updates. It's a quick and efficient way to stay informed about current events and trends.

5. Professional Networking: Virtual connections are valuable for professional networking and career development. Platforms like LinkedIn help individuals connect with potential employers, colleagues, and industry professionals.

6. Support Communities: Online support communities and forums provide a platform for individuals facing similar challenges or interests to connect and seek advice or solace.

Physical Connections:

1. In-Person Interaction: Physical connections involve face-to-face interaction with others. These connections are established through personal meetings, gatherings, and shared physical experiences.

2. Deeper Emotional Bonds: Physical connections often lead to deeper emotional bonds. In-person interactions allow people to read non-verbal cues, making it easier to connect on an emotional level.

3. Quality Time: Physical connections provide opportunities for quality time spent together. Shared experiences, such as travel, adventures, or simply being in the same physical space, can lead to lasting memories.

4. Haptic Communication: Physical connections allow for haptic communication, which involves touch and physical gestures. These forms of communication can convey empathy and support.

5. Spontaneity: In-person connections offer spontaneity and serendipity. Chance encounters and impromptu gatherings create opportunities for unexpected and memorable experiences.

6. Sense of Presence: Physical connections reinforce a sense of presence. Being physically present with others strengthens the feeling of belonging and togetherness.

Challenges and Balance:

Balancing virtual and physical connections is essential. Virtual connections can sometimes lack the depth and authenticity of in-person interactions, and they may lead to issues such as online harassment and disconnection. On the other hand, physical connections can be limited by geographical constraints and busy schedules.

Ultimately, the ideal balance between virtual and physical connections varies for each individual. A mix of both can provide a comprehensive social network, enabling individuals to stay connected to a wide range of people while also nurturing deeper, face-to-face relationships with those they hold most dear. The choice between virtual and physical connections depends on personal preferences, needs, and circumstances.

CHAPTER EIGHT

Longevity Around the World

In our global quest for the elixir of a long and joyful life, it's imperative to embark on a journey that transcends borders and encompasses diverse cultures, traditions, and practices. Chapter 9, "Longevity Around the World," is an expedition into the remarkable tapestry of human longevity, taking us across continents and oceans to explore the secrets and commonalities that bind us as inhabitants of this extraordinary planet. As we delve into the vibrant landscapes of longevity, you'll discover that the desire for a fulfilling and extended life is universal. While the pursuit of well-being may take on unique flavors and expressions in different corners of the world, the fundamental principles and values that guide us toward longevity are surprisingly consistent. From the serene island of Okinawa, Japan, to the bustling streets of Loma Linda, California, and the idyllic hills of Sardinia, Italy, we'll unravel the diverse practices and lifestyles that underpin the long and joyful lives of the world's centenarians. Through the lens of culture, diet, community, and purpose, we'll learn the lessons these global treasures offer and the profound wisdom they share. In this chapter, we'll venture into the heart of longevity hotspots, and with each step, we'll gain insights that can inspire and guide us toward a more vibrant and enduring existence. So, fasten your seatbelts, dear readers, as we embark on a world tour of wisdom and well-being, exploring the splendid mosaic of longevity that humanity has to offer. Together, we'll unearth the secrets and stories that unite us in our shared quest for a life rich in both years and joy.

Blue zones are known for longevity

Okinawa is one of the world's renowned Blue Zones, a region recognized for having a high concentration of centenarians, people who live to be 100 years old or older. Okinawa, a picturesque island located in Japan, has attracted the attention of researchers and health enthusiasts for its remarkable longevity and exceptional quality of life. Here's an explanation of Okinawa as a Blue Zone:

Okinawa as a Blue Zone:

1. Exceptional Longevity: Okinawa is celebrated for its exceptionally high life expectancy. The region boasts one of the world's highest concentrations of centenarians, and many Okinawans enjoy not just longer lives but also a higher quality of life in their later years.

2. Dietary Traditions: The Okinawan diet is often credited as a primary factor contributing to the region's longevity. It is characterized by a variety of nutrient-rich, plant-based foods, including sweet potatoes, tofu, seaweed, and an abundance of vegetables. The diet is typically low in calories but high in essential nutrients.

3. Active Lifestyles: Okinawans are known for their active lifestyles, and they engage in physical activities such as gardening, walking, and traditional forms of exercise well into their old age. Staying physically active is a key component of their longevity.

4. Strong Sense of Community: Okinawa places a strong emphasis on community bonds and social support. The concept of "moai" represents social groups that provide emotional and practical assistance, ensuring that individuals are surrounded by friends and support networks throughout their lives.

5. Cultural Practices: The cultural values and traditions of Okinawa, such as a sense of purpose, resilience, and respect for elders, contribute to the well-being and longevity of its residents.

6. Healthy Mindset: A positive outlook on life and a reduced sense of stress are also associated with Okinawan longevity. These psychological factors are thought to play a crucial role in overall well-being.

Okinawa serves as a compelling case study for researchers and health experts seeking to understand the secrets of long and healthy lives. Its residents exemplify a holistic approach to well-being, one that combines a nutrient-rich diet, physical activity, strong social connections, and a positive mindset. Okinawa's Blue Zone status underscores the idea that a balanced lifestyle can lead to extended years of vibrant and joyful living, and it offers valuable insights for anyone seeking to improve their health and longevity.

Sardinia is another well-known Blue Zone, recognized for its remarkable longevity and high concentration of centenarians. Sardinia, a large Italian island located in the Mediterranean Sea, has captured the attention of researchers and health enthusiasts for its unique cultural and lifestyle factors that contribute to the longevity of its residents. Here's an explanation of Sardinia as a Blue Zone:

Sardinia as a Blue Zone:

1. High Life Expectancy: Sardinia is celebrated for its high life expectancy, with a significant portion of its population living well into their 90s and 100s. This longevity is attributed to various lifestyle and environmental factors.

2. Traditional Sardinian Diet: The Sardinian diet is often considered one of the keys to longevity. It includes whole grains, legumes, olive oil, local vegetables, and goat's milk and cheese. These foods are rich in antioxidants and nutrients, contributing to overall health and well-being.

3. Physical Activity: The Sardinian lifestyle encourages physical activity through daily routines, such as tending to gardens, walking, and engaging in outdoor work. Regular exercise and an active way of life are essential components of Sardinians' longevity.

4. Strong Family and Community Ties: Sardinia places a strong emphasis on family and community bonds. Multigenerational households are common, and social support from close-knit communities is an integral part of Sardinian life.

5. Cultural Traditions: Sardinia's cultural practices, including rituals and celebrations, contribute to a sense of purpose, belonging, and mental well-being. These traditions foster positive mental health and emotional resilience.

6. Low-Stress Levels: Sardinia is known for its low-stress lifestyle. The relaxed pace of life, sense of community, and strong family ties help residents manage stress and maintain a more positive outlook.

7. Genetics and Isolation: Some researchers believe that a unique genetic makeup, along with the isolation of the island, may contribute to the exceptional longevity observed in Sardinia.

Sardinia serves as a fascinating case study for understanding the relationship between lifestyle, culture, and longevity. The island's residents exemplify the idea that a combination of a nutrient-rich diet, regular physical activity, strong social connections, cultural traditions, and a low-stress environment can contribute to a long and healthy life. Sardinia's Blue Zone status underscores the importance of holistic well-being and offers valuable insights for those seeking to improve their quality of life and longevity.

The Nicoya Peninsula is a prominent Blue Zone, recognized for its high life expectancy and a substantial population of centenarians. Located in Costa Rica, this stunning region has garnered attention for its unique lifestyle and cultural practices that contribute to the longevity of its residents. Here's an explanation of the Nicoya Peninsula as a Blue Zone:

Nicoya Peninsula as a Blue Zone:

1. Exceptional Life Expectancy: The Nicoya Peninsula is known for its high life expectancy, with a significant portion of its population living well into its 90s and beyond. This longevity is linked to specific lifestyle and cultural factors.

2. Healthy Diet: The Nicoyan diet is based on natural and unprocessed foods, including beans, corn, rice, tropical fruits, and local vegetables. These foods are rich in essential nutrients and contribute to overall health.

3. Daily Physical Activity: The people of the Nicoya Peninsula maintain active lives through activities like farming, fishing, and walking. Regular exercise and physical labor are integral to the region's longevity.

4. Strong Social Bonds: Nicoyans place a strong emphasis on family and community connections. Extended families often live together, and social support from close-knit communities plays a vital role in their well-being.

5. Cultural Traditions: Cultural practices and traditions, such as celebrations and social gatherings, create a sense of belonging, purpose, and mental well-being in the Nicoyan community.

6. Low-Stress Lifestyle: The Nicoya Peninsula is known for its low-stress lifestyle. The tranquil environment, strong community ties, and social support contribute to lower stress levels and a more positive outlook.

7. Clean Environment: The region benefits from clean air, uncontaminated water sources, and natural landscapes. These environmental factors support overall health and well-being.

The Nicoya Peninsula's status as a Blue Zone exemplifies the idea that a combination of a healthy, plant-based diet, regular physical activity, strong social connections, cultural traditions, a low-stress environment, and a clean natural setting can lead to long and healthy lives. The region offers valuable insights for those interested in improving their quality of life and longevity by adopting a holistic approach to well-being.

Ikaria, a Greek island in the Aegean Sea, is recognized as a Blue Zone, a region known for having a high concentration of centenarians and a population that enjoys remarkable longevity and well-being. Here's an explanation of Ikaria as a Blue Zone:

Ikaria as a Blue Zone:

1. High Life Expectancy: Ikaria is celebrated for its high life expectancy, with a notable proportion of its population living well into their 90s and even surpassing the age of 100. This exceptional longevity is attributed to a combination of lifestyle and environmental factors.

2. Mediterranean Diet: The Ikarian diet is largely influenced by the Mediterranean diet, which includes olive oil, whole grains, vegetables, legumes, and an abundance of locally grown herbs. This diet is known for its health-promoting properties and contributes to overall well-being.

3. Active Lifestyles: Ikarians are known for their active lives, as they often engage in daily activities like walking, gardening, and tending to their land. Physical activity is a central aspect of their longevity.

4. Strong Community Bonds: The residents of Ikaria emphasize strong family and community bonds. Close-knit communities and social support networks play a vital role in their well-being.

5. Cultural Traditions: Cultural practices and traditions, including celebrations and festivals, foster a sense of purpose, community, and mental well-being among the island's residents.

6. Low-Stress Levels: Ikaria is renowned for its low-stress lifestyle. The island's peaceful environment, close social connections, and the influence of the Mediterranean way of life contribute to reduced stress levels and a positive mindset.

7. Natural Environment: Ikaria's natural environment, with its clean air, access to nature, and tranquil landscapes, supports overall health and well-being.

Ikaria serves as a captivating example of how a combination of a nutritious diet, regular physical activity, strong social connections, cultural traditions, low stress, and a pristine natural setting can lead to a long and vibrant life. The island's status as a Blue Zone underscores the importance of embracing a holistic approach to well-being and offers valuable insights for those looking to enhance their quality of life and longevity.

Loma Linda, a city in California, is a unique Blue Zone in the United States, known for its high life expectancy and a population that enjoys remarkable longevity and overall well-being. Here's an explanation of Loma Linda as a Blue Zone:

Loma Linda as a Blue Zone:

1. Notable Longevity: Loma Linda is celebrated for its high life expectancy, with a significant portion of its population living well into their 90s and beyond. This exceptional longevity is associated with lifestyle and cultural factors.

2. Plant-Based Diet: One of the distinguishing features of Loma Linda's Blue Zone is its emphasis on a plant-based diet. Many residents follow a vegetarian or vegan lifestyle, focusing on whole grains, legumes, nuts, and an abundance of fruits and vegetables. This diet is rich in nutrients and contributes to overall well-being.

3. Healthy Lifestyles: Loma Linda residents are committed to a health-conscious lifestyle that includes regular exercise, access to nature, and participation in outdoor activities. These practices promote physical well-being and contribute to their longevity.

4. Strong Social Bonds: The community of Loma Linda places a strong emphasis on close-knit social bonds. Family, faith-based connections, and social support networks play a significant role in the well-being of its residents.

5. Cultural Traditions: The community's cultural and religious practices, many of which involve healthy living and social engagement, contribute to a sense of purpose and mental well-being among its residents.

6. Low-Stress Lifestyle: Loma Linda is known for its low-stress lifestyle. The combination of a peaceful environment, strong social connections, and a health-conscious way of life contributes to lower stress levels and a positive mindset.

7. Faith and Spirituality: Many Loma Linda residents are part of the Seventh-day Adventist faith, which emphasizes healthy living and overall well-being as a fundamental part of its beliefs.

Loma Linda's status as a Blue Zone underscores the importance of a holistic approach to well-being. It serves as an example of how embracing a plant-based diet, regular physical activity, strong social connections, cultural traditions, low stress, and faith-based values can lead to a long and fulfilling life. The city offers valuable insights for those seeking to improve their quality of life and longevity by adopting a comprehensive approach to well-being.

Cultural practices that contribute to longevity are the traditional behaviors, rituals, and customs of specific communities or regions that have been linked to longer and healthier lives. These practices are often deeply ingrained in the daily lives of individuals and have been passed down through generations. Here are some examples of cultural practices that promote longevity:

1. Dietary Traditions: Many cultures have dietary practices that emphasize the consumption of nutrient-rich, whole foods. For instance, the Mediterranean diet, which includes olive oil, fruits, vegetables, and lean proteins, has been associated with better health and longevity. Similarly, the Japanese practice of eating a variety of fresh, seasonal, and locally sourced foods, such as seafood and vegetables, has contributed to the longevity of the Okinawan population.

2. Fasting and Caloric Restriction: Some cultures incorporate periodic fasting or caloric restriction as part of their religious or cultural practices. These practices have been shown to have potential health benefits, including improved metabolic health and increased longevity.

3. Social Cohesion: Cultures that prioritize strong social bonds and community support tend to have lower stress levels and improved mental health. Social gatherings, family reunions, and community events play a significant role in promoting longevity in such cultures.

4. Physical Activity: Many cultures incorporate regular physical activity into their daily routines. This can include practices like gardening, walking, dancing, and engaging in manual labor. Consistent physical activity supports better physical health and longevity.

5. Cultural Values: Cultural values related to respect for elders, wisdom, and social support are often associated with better overall well-being and longevity. In some cultures, older individuals are highly respected and actively involved in the community.

6. Religious and Spiritual Practices: Many cultures have strong religious or spiritual practices that provide a sense of purpose and meaning in life. These practices can promote mental and emotional well-being, reducing stress and contributing to a longer life.

7. Herbal Remedies and Traditional Medicine: Some cultures have a rich tradition of using herbal remedies and traditional forms of medicine to promote health and prevent illness. These practices can support physical well-being and longevity.

8. Stress Reduction Techniques: Certain cultural practices emphasize stress reduction and relaxation through activities like meditation, deep breathing, or mindfulness. These practices help individuals manage stress and maintain better mental health.

9. Cultural Celebrations and Rituals: Cultural celebrations, rituals, and ceremonies often involve dancing, music, and physical activity. These events bring communities together and provide an opportunity for physical and emotional expression.

10. Healthy Aging Traditions: Some cultures have specific traditions and rituals that celebrate and encourage healthy aging. These practices may include specific foods, ceremonies, or activities that support well-being in later life.

Cultural practices that promote longevity are a testament to the diverse ways in which different societies have recognized and celebrated the importance of living long and fulfilling lives. These practices often reflect the wisdom and knowledge of the community and serve as a source of inspiration for those seeking to improve their health and well-being.

Scientific insights into longevity are findings and research conclusions that help us better understand the biological, physiological, and environmental factors that influence how long individuals live and the quality of their lives. Scientists have uncovered numerous insights into longevity by studying various aspects of human biology, genetics, lifestyle, and environmental influences. Here are some key scientific insights into longevity:

1. Genetics and Longevity: Genetic factors play a significant role in determining an individual's potential for a long life. Certain genes are associated with a decreased risk of age-related diseases and longer lifespans. These genetic insights have led to the identification of "longevity genes" that influence factors like cellular repair and immune system function.

2. Cellular Aging: Research has revealed that the rate of cellular aging and the stability of DNA can impact longevity. Telomeres, protective caps at the ends of chromosomes, have been linked to aging. Shortened telomeres are associated with a higher risk of age-related diseases.

3. Nutrition and Caloric Restriction: Caloric restriction and specific dietary patterns have been shown to extend lifespan and reduce the risk of age-related diseases. These insights have contributed to the study of the molecular mechanisms behind caloric restriction's positive effects on longevity.

4. Inflammation and Chronic Disease: Chronic inflammation is linked to many age-related diseases. Scientific research has shown that lifestyle factors, such as diet and physical activity, can reduce inflammation, leading to improved health and longevity.

5. Cellular Repair Mechanisms: Understanding how cells repair damage and maintain their integrity has provided insights into the aging process. Enhancing cellular repair and autophagy (the process of removing damaged cells) may contribute to longevity.

6. Hormonal Regulation: Hormonal balance is vital for healthy aging. Scientific research has led to insights into the effects of hormones like growth hormone, insulin-like growth factor 1 (IGF-1), and sex hormones on the aging process.

7. Brain Health: Cognitive health is an integral part of aging. Insights into brain health have highlighted the importance of maintaining cognitive function and preventing conditions like Alzheimer's disease. Brain exercises, social engagement, and a healthy diet can contribute to a longer and more fulfilling life.

8. Exercise and Physical Activity: Scientific studies consistently show that regular physical activity is associated with better physical health, mental well-being, and a longer life. Understanding the physiological benefits of exercise has led to the promotion of active lifestyles for longevity.

9. Mental and Emotional Well-Being: Research into the connection between mental health, stress reduction, and longevity has highlighted the importance of

positive emotional states. Stress management, mindfulness, and social support are linked to a longer and healthier life.

10. Environmental Factors: Insights into the impact of environmental factors such as air quality, access to green spaces, and clean water have underlined the importance of living in a supportive and healthy environment for longevity.

11. Quality of Healthcare: Advances in medical science, including early disease detection, improved treatments, and preventive measures, have had a significant impact on increasing lifespans.

12. Social Connections and Community: The influence of strong social connections and a sense of belonging on mental and physical health is well-documented. Research shows that people with robust social networks tend to live longer and healthier lives.

Scientific insights into longevity continue to evolve as researchers delve deeper into the complex interplay of genetics, biology, lifestyle, and environment. These insights provide valuable knowledge that can inform lifestyle choices, medical practices, and public health policies, ultimately contributing to a longer and healthier life for individuals and populations.

Conclusion: The Global Pursuit of Longevity

In the enthralling exploration of "Longevity Around the World," we embarked on a captivating journey through the diverse landscapes of human existence. This chapter, titled "By Being OK," unraveled the secrets and wisdom that bind us as inhabitants of this extraordinary planet. Our global quest for a long and joyful life took us from the serene islands of Okinawa to the bustling streets of Loma Linda, and from the idyllic hills of Sardinia to the vibrant communities of the Nicoya Peninsula and the enchanting island of Ikaria.

As we roamed these longevity hotspots, it became abundantly clear that the desire for a fulfilling and extended life is universal. While the practices and traditions that guide us toward longevity may take on unique flavors in different corners of the world, the fundamental principles and values that underlie our shared quest for a vibrant existence remain remarkably consistent.

From the pages of this chapter, we have learned that the path to a long and joyful life is woven into the tapestry of culture, diet, community, and purpose. Whether it's the balanced diet of Okinawa, the familial bonds of Sardinia, the active lifestyles of the Nicoya Peninsula, the Mediterranean magic of Ikaria, or the faith-based health consciousness of Loma Linda, each culture has provided us with profound insights.

In this culminating chapter, "By Being Ok," we discovered that true longevity transcends the simple addition of years. It resides in the profound understanding that life, no matter where it's lived, is most enriched by quality over quantity. The pursuit of well-being, informed by cultural practices, shared traditions, and scientific insights, teaches us that to live long and joyfully, one must nurture the mind, body, and spirit.

Our global journey through these remarkable longevity hotspots has offered invaluable lessons and universal truths. It has shown us that, ultimately, the path to a long and joyful life is not confined by borders, but rather illuminated by the shared human experience. As we conclude our exploration of "Longevity Around the World," we carry with us the wisdom and hope that the pursuit of well-being is a journey we all share, irrespective of our place on the map, and that by being "okay," we can find the keys to lasting health and happiness.

CHAPTER NINE
Conclusion and Preparing for a Long and Joyful Life

In this opening chapter, we embark on a voyage into the profound exploration of a life filled with purpose, fulfillment, and boundless joy. Life is a journey, and how we navigate it shapes our destinies. This book will serve as your compass, guiding you through the seas of existence, and offering insights, tools, and wisdom to help you chart a course towards a long and joyful life. Together, we will discover the keys to not only prolonging our time on this planet but also savoring every moment of it. So, prepare to embark on this adventure, for the voyage of a lifetime awaits.

The "American Fountain of Youth" is a metaphorical concept that symbolizes the idea of maintaining youthfulness, vitality, and a high quality of life as one grows older. It draws inspiration from the mythical Fountain of Youth, which, according to legends, had the power to restore youth and grant immortality to those who drank from it.

In the context of your book, "American Fountain of Youth" represents a mindset and a way of living that can help individuals achieve a long and joyful life. Here are some key aspects of the power of the "American Fountain of Youth":

1. Positive Aging: It encourages individuals to embrace the process of aging with a positive attitude. Instead of fearing or resisting getting older, the concept promotes the idea that aging can be a rewarding experience.

2. Health and Wellness: The "American Fountain of Youth" emphasizes the importance of maintaining good physical and mental health through a healthy lifestyle. This includes aspects like proper nutrition, regular exercise, and stress management.

3. Mindset and Attitude: A youthful mindset is seen as a powerful tool for longevity and happiness. It encourages people to maintain a curious, open-minded, and optimistic outlook on life.

4.*Pursuit of Passions: Engaging in activities that one is passionate about is considered a vital component of the "American Fountain of Youth." It's about finding joy and purpose in one's hobbies, interests, and creative endeavors.

5. Social Connections: Building and nurturing positive relationships with others is believed to be a key to a joyful life. This includes maintaining strong connections with family and friends and fostering a sense of community and belonging.

6. Adaptability: The concept promotes adaptability and resilience in the face of life's challenges. It suggests that those who can adapt to change and learn from their experiences are more likely to lead fulfilling lives.

7. Life-Long Learning: Continuous learning and personal growth are valued elements of the "American Fountain of Youth." It encourages individuals to stay curious and continue acquiring new knowledge and skills.

8. Giving Back: Contributing to the well-being of others and giving back to the community is seen as a source of fulfillment. It suggests that acts of kindness and philanthropy can add meaning to one's life.

In essence, the "American Fountain of Youth" is a way of life that focuses on proactively nurturing physical, mental, and emotional well-being while maintaining a positive and purposeful mindset. It's not about seeking eternal youth but about aging gracefully and joyfully, making the most of each stage of life. This concept reminds individuals that they have the power to shape their aging journey and live a fulfilling life, regardless of their age.

The promise of a joyful life is a powerful and optimistic vision of what life can be when one consciously pursues happiness, fulfillment, and contentment. It's the idea that by making deliberate choices and adopting certain attitudes and behaviors, individuals can significantly enhance their overall quality of life. Here are some key elements that constitute the promise of a joyful life:

1. Happiness and Contentment: At the heart of this promise is the pursuit of happiness and contentment. It acknowledges that true joy comes from within and can be cultivated through positive thoughts, experiences, and relationships.

2. Purpose and Meaning: A joyful life often involves a sense of purpose and meaning. It's about feeling that one's life has value and that one's actions and contributions matter.

3. Positive Relationships:* Strong, supportive, and loving relationships with family and friends are essential for a joyful life. These connections provide emotional support, companionship, and a sense of belonging.

4. Gratitude: Practicing gratitude and appreciating the small and big blessings in life is a fundamental aspect of a joyful life. Gratitude helps shift focus away from what's lacking and toward what's present and positive.

5. Fulfilling Activities: Engaging in activities, hobbies, or work that one is passionate about can bring immense joy. These pursuits provide a sense of accomplishment and personal satisfaction.

6.*Emotional Resilience:*The ability to bounce back from adversity and cope with life's challenges is crucial for a joyful life. Resilience helps individuals maintain a positive outlook, even in difficult times.

7. Self-Care: Taking care of one's physical and mental health is part of the promise of a joyful life. Self-care practices, such as exercise, meditation, and relaxation, contribute to overall well-being.

8. Balance: Achieving a balance between various aspects of life, such as work, leisure, and personal time, is important for happiness. A balanced life allows for personal growth and enjoyment.

9. Optimism: An optimistic outlook on life can help individuals overcome obstacles and view setbacks as opportunities for growth.

10. Continuous Learning: A commitment to lifelong learning and personal growth is a hallmark of a joyful life. It fosters a sense of curiosity and self-improvement.

11. Kindness and Generosity: Acts of kindness and generosity, whether toward others or oneself, are associated with increased happiness and a sense of fulfillment.

12. Living in the Present: The promise of a joyful life often encourages individuals to be fully present in the moment, rather than dwelling on the past or worrying about the future.

In essence, the promise of a joyful life is a belief that individuals have the power to shape their happiness and fulfillment. It's a commitment to making choices and cultivating habits that lead to a life filled with positivity, purpose, and well-being. While challenges and difficulties may arise, the promise of a joyful life suggests that with the right mindset and actions, one can navigate life's ups and downs with grace and resilience.

Wisdom Words:

"Embrace the gift of each day with a heart full of gratitude, a mind open to learning, and a spirit eager to share kindness. In these simple yet profound acts, you'll uncover the secret to a lifetime of joy."

Call to Action:

"*As you close this book and embark on your journey towards a long and joyful life, remember that the power to shape your destiny lies within you. I encourage you to take the following actions today:*

1. Set Clear Goals: Define your aspirations and set achievable goals for your future. Write them down and create a plan to work towards them.

2. *Practice Gratitude:* Start a daily gratitude journal. Write down three things you're grateful for each day, no matter how small or significant.

3. *Nurture Relationships: Reach out to a loved one you haven't connected with in a while. Strengthen your bonds with family and friends.*

4. *Engage in a Passion: Dedicate time to a hobby or interest that brings you joy. Rekindle your passions.*

5. *Take Care of Your Health:* Commit to a healthier lifestyle. Incorporate regular exercise and balanced nutrition into your daily routine.

6. *Learn Something New: Identify a subject or skill you've always wanted to explore and take the first steps toward learning it.*

7. *Give Back: Find a way to give back to your community or a cause you're passionate about. Acts of kindness make a difference.*

8. *Stay Present Practice mindfulness. Spend a few moments each day living in the present, appreciating the beauty of now.*

Remember*, a joyful life is not a destination but a continuous journey. Seize each day as an opportunity to shape your destiny and find happiness in the smallest of moments. Your life is your masterpiece, and you are the artist. Paint it with the vibrant colors of joy, purpose, and fulfillment."*